Restored Harmony **Reviews**

"…this book is a fine and eloquent combination of modern science, ancient wisdom, and practical guidance, literate and accessible, as well as scientifically sound. I recommend it to all those who are concerned with creating more effective, humane, and comprehensive programs of cancer care."

James S. Gordon, M.D.
Director, The Center for Mind-Body Medicine, Washington DC;
Clinical Professor, Georgetown University School of Medicine; Chair of the White House Commission on
Complementary and Alternative Medicine Policy.

———————— ☯ ————————

"This book is compelling reading for all those who look after cancer patients, regardless of whether they are healthcare professionals or lay family members. Cancer victims will also find it helpful and encouraging, and even 'hard nosed' researchers, like myself, can learn a great deal from it".

Edzard Ernst M.D. Ph.D. F.R.C.P. (Edin.),
Professor, Department of Complementary Medicine,
School of Sport and Health Sciences,
University of Exeter, United Kingdom.
Author of Complementary and Alternative Medicine: A Desktop Reference.

———————— ☯ ————————

"Restored Harmony skillfully blends Eastern and Western approaches to cancer in this compelling overview of the fascinating relationships emerging between Traditional Chinese Medicine, immunotherapy, psycho-neuro-oncology, complexity theory, and quantum physics. Dr. Sagar takes us on an inspired, thoughtful journey into mind-body medicine of the future."

John Boik MAcOM,
Author of Natural Compounds in Cancer Therapy

———————— ☯ ————————

"Stephen Sagar MD creates a symphony from the cacophony that cancer often creates. He shows how prevention of disease and restoration of the harmony of health can be achieved by correctly blending the advice of conventional and Traditional Chinese Medicine. As a result, we are blessed with an enlightened insider's view of cancer and its treatment".

Mehmet Oz MD, MBA
Irving Assistant Professor of Surgery in the Division of Cardiac Surgery
at Columbia University in New York. Director of the cardiac assist device program and the
complementary medicine program at Columbia Presbyterian Medical Center.
Author of Healing from the Heart.

Restored Harmony:

An Evidence Based Approach for Integrating Traditional Chinese Medicine into Complementary Cancer Care

Stephen M. Sagar MD

Dreaming DragonFly Communications
Hamilton, Ontario

Catalogued in the National Library of Canada

ISBN: 0-9689488-0-4 (paperback)
1. Cancer
2. Traditional Chinese Medicine
3. Mind-Body Medicine

Graphic Design, photography and final production
by Christina M. Garchinski.

Printing Services: J. H. French & Co.

First printing October 2001.

Dreaming DragonFly Communications™ is a Canadian multimedia company with
a vision to improve healthcare and lifestyle. Book orders welcome. Contact us at
dragonflycom@home.com.

To my daughter, Natalie:
Thank you for your innocent wisdom.

And to my mother, Sheila:
You were courageous and loving to the very end.

Contents

Contents

Acknowledgements

The word 'inspire' is derived from spirit and can mean strength, courage and will, as well as to 'take a deep breath'. I was inspired when I first read 'Manifesto for a New Medicine' by James Gordon MD. I was subsequently delighted when Jim altruistically came to talk to us about the 'New Medicine' at an educational seminar on complementary medicine that I arranged in Toronto. I was further inspired and encouraged by Jim's energy, credibility and courage to discuss territories that are normally out of bounds for conventional medicine. I was thrilled to be accepted into the Center for Mind-Body Medicine's professional training programs. From then on, Jim has become a close professional colleague, friend and mentor, and I have been privileged to be part of the planning committee for the annual Comprehensive Cancer Care Conferences, and a member of the teaching faculty for the successful Cancer Guides Course. Jim has literally inspired and encouraged me to further implement my vision for a more patient-orientated medicine that recognizes the integration of the mind and body, the reality of spirit, and the pioneering soul of science to push forward the frontiers of medicine into new realms, such as consciousness and quantum physics. The philosophy of Traditional Chinese Medicine contributes the foundations of Mind-Body Medicine, recognizes energy and spirit, and curiously contains the elements of modern physics. Thank you Jim for your encouragement, generosity of time, and writing the foreword for this book.

I wish to thank John Boik, Edzard Ernst, Henry Dreher, Esther Sternberg, and Ralph Moss for reviewing the manuscript of this book. John Boik has contributed vastly to our current knowledge of Chinese herbal preparations and anti-cancer therapy and I highly recommend his new book, 'Natural Compounds in Cancer Therapy'. Edzard Ernst is professor of Complementary Medicine at the University of Exeter and a leading authority for the application of evidence-based medicine to complementary and alternative therapies (CAM). He is responsible for the journal, 'Focus on Alternative and Complementary Therapies', that has set a high standard for sorting out the wheat from the chaff in CAM. I recommend his recent book, 'Complementary and Alternative Medicine: A Desktop Reference'. Henry Dreher is a pioneer in the education and development of mind-body medicine and has written numerous books and articles on psycho-neuro-immunology (PNI) and health. He is also a Cancer Guide, helping patients to seek information and make decisions when evaluating therapeutic programs. Esther Sternberg directs the Behavioral Integrative Neuroscience Program at the National Institute of Mental Health and is a leader in research on emotions, health and disease. She has written an eloquent book entitled, 'The Balance Within', that discusses the science of PNI, and discusses links between our current scientific concepts and ancient philosophies of healthcare. Ralph Moss has courageously been a critic of the conventional way we approach cancer treatment and has stimulated much discussion towards the new directions we must take to improve patient care and to evaluate novel therapies. Ralph has published numerous scientific books on unconventional cancer therapies.

Thank you Raimond Wong MD, my esteemed professional colleague and friend at the Hamilton Regional Cancer Centre. Together, we form a critical mass of radiation oncologists who use TCM in clinical practice. We have had many fruitful discussions and initiated several studies to evaluate TCM in a conventional cancer clinic.

Thank you to all my patients who have taught me so much more than medical school or books.

Lastly, thank you to my parents, David and Sheila Sagar for all the subtle contributions in early life that directed me to where I am now. My mother's untimely death from pancreatic cancer was both a tragedy and an inspiration for my further growth.

Preface

By Edzard Ernst MD, PhD, FRCP

There is no shortage of books on complementary medicine. In fact, I sometimes get the impression that more books than scientific investigations of this area are presently being published. But Stephen Sagar's book clearly stands out from this somewhat confusing plethora of writing. It takes an approach that is unusual, inspired and strangely convincing. Dr. Sagar's aim is obviously not to sum up the latest scientific knowledge, neither does this author fall into the trap of so many before him, namely to blindly promote certain therapeutic approaches on the basis of usually flimsy evidence.

Dr. Sagar unpretentiously takes his readers on a journey. The sites on this journey are concepts of ancient Chinese medicine, narratives of patients, modern medical science, art, wisdom, and humanity. The destination of this journey is a new type of cancer care that is holistic in the best sense of the word. Thanks to the vast experience and exceptional skills of Dr. Sagar, the journey is not only pleasant but widens the mind and instils hope.

This book is compelling reading for all those who look after cancer patients, regardless of whether they are healthcare professionals or lay family members. Cancer victims will also find it helpful and encouraging, and even 'hard nosed' researchers, like myself, can learn a great deal from it.

Edzard Ernst M.D. Ph.D. F.R.C.P. (Edin.),
*Professor, Department of Complementary Medicine,
School of Sport and Health Sciences,
University of Exeter, United Kingdom.*

Author of Complementary and Alternative Medicine:
A Desktop Reference.

Foreword

By James Gordon MD

Over the last twenty years, I've been exploring the integration of Chinese medicine into individualized programs of comprehensive care for cancer patients. Each year, at the Comprehensive Cancer Care Conferences of the Center for Mind-Body Medicine, we hear about the latest research on these therapies, in the West as well as in China. It is now clear to me and to many others in the field, that Chinese medicine can, and should, be available to everyone who is being treated for cancer.

This new book, by Dr. Stephen Sagar, makes this case in a way that is at once evidence-based, thoughtful and poetic. Dr. Sagar is a radiation oncologist who deals every day with the challenges of cancer treatment, and with the accompanying side-effects of treatment. He is a fine clinical observer and an imaginative, indeed, visionary thinker. What he has done in this brief book is to describe precisely and well the worldview of the 4000-year-old Chinese medicine, and how its traditional approach to cancer treatment may dovetail with our most modern western scientific understanding and technological approaches.

Dr. Sagar understands the power of Chinese therapies – acupuncture, herbal therapies, the exercises of Qi Gong, hands on healing, and above all, intention. He shows us how these therapies are already being used to enhance immunity, improve overall physiological functioning, frustrate tumor growth, improve mood, and provide relief for such debilitating treatment side-effects as nausea, vomiting, pain, fatigue, diarrhea, and mouth ulcers. He shares with us the modern scientific papers on which his conclusions are based, and lets us know when evidence is lacking. Equally importantly, he gives us a sense of

Chinese medicine, and of how it may well contribute in significant ways to the more harmonious functioning of our minds and our spirit, as well as our bodies.

In summary, this book is a fine and eloquent combination of modern science, ancient wisdom, and practical guidance, literate and accessible, as well as scientifically sound. I recommend it to all those who are concerned with creating more effective, humane, and comprehensive programs of cancer care.

James S. Gordon, M.D.
Director, The Center for Mind-Body Medicine, Washington DC;
Clinical Professor, Georgetown University School of Medicine;
Chair of the White House Commission on Complementary and
Alternative Medicine Policy;

Co-author, Comprehensive Cancer Care: Integrating
Complementary, Alternative, and Conventional Therapies.

Introduction

My interest in Traditional Chinese Medicine was fueled by a fascination of the intricate and sophisticated relationships between the mind, body and the environment, concepts that are surely lacking in current, conventional medicine. I excelled in biology at high school, and my graduate background was in pharmacology. As an adolescent, I was both a mystic and a scientist-in-training. I was intrigued by the dynamic symphony of molecular interactions that were associated with life. As a mystic, how could I integrate the concept of vitalism with science. Is it possible to combine magic and science?

During my arduous training as a physician, many of these mystical concepts were drummed out of me by our boot camp system of medical training. Yet when I practiced medicine, I was not dealing with a reductionist collection of molecules, but a whole person consisting of a unique soul driven by spirit, and subject to all the infirmities of the physical world. The person was much more than the anatomical structure we were taught at medical school. The person is a unique system of memories, emotions, relationships, and *individual* responses. Many people live their lives through metaphorical representations of their environment. We are not necessarily logical creatures . We are a complex tapestry of our ancestors' genes and our own unique experiences. Moreover, we are changing and adapting, undergoing transitions, evolving and growing. These aspects of the human being seemed much more important to me than the dogmatic reductionist proposals that were often espoused by conventional medicine.

It will be apparent that it is difficult to discern which properties each thing possesses in reality
**Democritus,
8th Century BC.**

Yet, our current scientific and technological medical system provides some miraculous therapies when we are sick. I marvel at cancers dissolving after treatment with radiotherapy, the restoration to health of a sick child with leukemia through powerful chemotherapy drugs, and the surgical excision and cure of a malignant bowel tumor. So what is missing? The answer is found in alchemy. The ultimate system of medicine and healthcare is to be found by being open minded and building bridges between the different disciplines. We need to understand how our thought processes and emotions can influence the physical changes in our body. It is important to recognize that there *is* a potential healing connection between people. Prayer *can* help us get better. Our states of mind *can* be as powerful in the restoration of our health as certain drugs. We need to restore faith in the power of ourselves as human beings to heal, and to be healed. We need to recognize that we are all *unique* individuals, not simply an average extrapolation of the general population. In aiming for the alchemical 'philosophers stone' of healthcare, we need to recognize that we are spiritual beings in a human body. For some people, being a spiritual being may be just a metaphor, but it is a powerful one, all the same, and conjures up the mystical complexity that makes us human beings.

Traditional Chinese Medicine is a model that metaphorically and philosophically formulates many of the complexities of being a human being, that I thought were lacking from our conventional healthcare system in North America and Europe. My challenge is to articulate the underlying science that I believe justifies utilizing this philosophy as part of our technology-based healthcare system. My task is made a little easier by the recognition of modern scientific systems theories, the age of computers and information technology, quantum physics, and modern concepts of energy transfer. In addition, public opinion has driven the methodologists to develop ways of evaluating complementary therapies, including the so-called gold standard, the proverbial double blind randomized controlled trial. In addition, governments are now more likely to sponsor research into complementary and alternative medicine.

Exactness is a fake

Alfred North Whitehead (1861-1947).

I am confident that this is just the beginning of the evolution of a planetary healthcare system that will recognize the uniqueness of us, that is, human beings.

This book is aimed at all healthcare practitioners, especially those with an interest in cancer treatment. It is also of interest to people who have or who have had cancer, as well as members of their family. You could use this book as a platform for discussion with your physician or other healthcare practitioner, especially since it provides scientific references. Some of the material may appear naive to some healthcare 'experts' and some of the science may be sophisticated for the layman outside of medicine. However, the aim is to build bridges and to open up your minds to new possibilities, that may be appropriate to your patients' health, your own health, and the health of our whole society.

☯ *Chapter One*

The Philosophy and Science of Traditional Chinese Medicine

- Mind-Body Integration

- Individual Uniqueness

- Mind as In-formation Transfer

- Communication Systems

- The Power of Healing

- The Main Components of Traditional Chinese Medicine

- Chinese Herbs

- Acupuncture

- Manipulation of Energy Flow

- The Clinical Practice of Traditional Chinese Medicine

☯ *Mind-Body Integration*

Recent evidence suggests that many traditional Chinese medical therapies are scientifically effective for the supportive care of people with cancer. The holistic approach of Traditional Chinese Medicine (TCM) may be integrated into conventional Western Medicine to supplement deficiencies in the current biomedical model. The philosophy of TCM proposes novel hypotheses that will support the development of a science-based holistic medicine. What is missing from Western medicine is the holistic concept of functional harmony interweaving our body and mind. Perhaps this is incorporated in the word spirit. People who are sick from cancer and the side-effects of their treatment express a sense of fragmentation and depersonalization. It is as though the orchestral symphony of their life has fallen apart into disharmony. Even when the cancer is cured, many people are left in constitutional disarray, disconnected from their song of life. Does Chinese Medicine provide a theory that can be used to reassemble the harmony that constitutes the symphony of life? Can this be applied to modern scientific theory and methodology? Moreover, can we apply a combination of conventional oncology and TCM to enhance the cure of cancer, reduce side-effects, improve quality of life, plus restore the harmony of vitality and a sense of purpose that constitute the meaning of life? I believe that the intelligent integration of TCM into cancer care can enhance our cancer treatment programs and encourage a holistic model of healthcare practice.

> I have the conviction that when physiology will be far enough advanced, the poet, the philosopher, and the physiologist will all understand each other.
> *Claude Bernard (1813-1878)*

> Like everything else in nature, music is a becoming, and it becomes its full self, when its sounds and laws are used by intelligent man for the production of harmony, and so made the vehicle of emotion and thought.
> *Theodore Mungers*

Individual Uniqueness ☯

The beauty of TCM is that it recognizes the person as an individual with his or her own unique personality and genetic constitution. Although the diagnostic system of TCM recognizes certain *categories* of constitutional type, its practice emphasizes that no two individuals are alike. It provides a model that represents emotional expression through Organ systems, and provides a bridge between emotional charactcristics and physical health or sickness. Classically, anger is related to the Liver, anxiety and sorrow to the Lungs, obsessional thought to the Spleen, fear to the Kidneys, and joy or optimism to the Heart. For example, those individuals with a weak Kidney essence constitution, may be particularly susceptible to life-long fatigue and infections. An individual with an excess of Liver yang tends to easily become angry and may be susceptible to high blood pressure and cardiovascular disease. Repressed and internalized anger may be a factor in the development of some cancers. Spleen deficiency may result from excess rumination and be associated with digestive difficulties. Disturbance of the Heart or shen may be reflected by anxiety and insomnia. In other words, TCM emphasizes the connection between the emotions and physical outcome. It also recognizes that our constitution at birth, mainly genetically determined, and our personality-dependent coping skills, can precipitate the development of disease later in life. The objective of TCM is to rebalance a system that is not in harmony to protect our personal 'Achilles' heel'.

☯ *Mind as In-formation Transfer*

Although the ancient Chinese were presumably unaware of the biochemical and neurological connections between the nervous system, immunocytes, cell membranes, and the nucleic acids that form our genes, we now know scientifically that there are processes that enable all of our cells to talk to each other. Prior to the 17th century, most healthcare traditions perceived mind, body, and spirit as inseparable and part of a single process. Unfortunately, the philosopher Renée Descartes suggested that mind and body were separate entities, a philosophical system termed dualism. Scientific evidence suggests that mind and body are connected as one, but dualism became established for at least two centuries, more for political reasons than science, by Sir Francis Bacon, who wished to separate the functions of the Church and State. The Church became responsible for the mind or soul, whereas the scientists and the State controlled the body. We now know that there is an intimate connection between our experience of mind and the physiological functioning of our body. This more recent scientific evidence is applied clinically by clinicians who practice Mind-Body-Spirit Medicine. Our physical function and the way we perceive emotions, think, react, and cope, are all dynamically connected and influence each other. There is indeed good evidence that the processes which coordinate the growth, development and relationship of our cells are the components of our mind, that stretches from the unconscious to normal awareness. Certain experimental mind states, from meditation to hallucinogenic drugs, have revealed that we can be made aware of the processes of the mind-body network, even at the preconscious level. This new knowledge empowers us and enables us to be in the driving seat when we make wise decisions about our health. Current evidence suggests that being empowered with knowledge and being part of the decision-making process results in an improved health outcome, whereas passivity and perceived lack of control may be detrimental to health.

Breath is the bridge which connects life to consciousness, which unites your body to your thoughts.
Thich Nhat Hanh
Vietnamese Buddhist Monk

Communication Systems ☯

Chinese Medicine views the body-mind network as a series of inter-related systems. These are commonly referred to as Organ *systems* and are denoted by the following ten Organs: Large Intestine, Small Intestine, Stomach, Gall Bladder, Triple Warmer, Spleen, Heart, Pericardium, Kidney and Lung (note that in contrast to anatomical organs, these systems are represented by upper case letters). The Organ systems are represented by surface points that run along so-called meridians, that are channels that carry information within each system via energy flow. Anatomically, these may represent neurological pathways that lead to the control centers of the autonomic nervous system in the brain stem. There are also extra meridian pathways, including the Greater Vessel and Conception Vessel pathways that run midline down the back and up the front of the body, respectively. Together, these systems form a complex information transfer system that allows modulation of the mind-body connection. Manipulation of these systems can readjust emotions, control neurological activity and neurotransmitter release, modulate hormone levels, change blood flow, influence the activity of immune cells and then ultimately, can influence genetic expression and cell proliferation.

☯ *The Power of Healing*

Chinese Medicine utilizes a variety of tools to manipulate the mind-body systems. Firstly, an expert practitioner of TCM will recognize that maximum healing occurs with the practitioner's intent to benefit the patient. The effect of this healing intent has a scientific basis that will be discussed later in this book. Sending healing messages to the person to be healed is well-described in recent research on prayer. The information transfer from healer to patient may be through the quantum-based theory of non-local energy transfer, or through entrainment of the patient's electromagnetic (EM) field by the EM field of the practitioner's own heart. The process of regulating the beat-to-beat variation of the heart (associated with loving-intent, calmness and focus) is termed 'centering' by therapeutic touch practitioners, and compassionate or loving kindness (metta) meditation by Buddhists. Cardiac entrainment influences the autonomic or 'involuntary' nervous system that, in turn, can influence cell behavior directly or through hormones and immunocytes. Giving hope, belief, acceptance and faith, when appropriate, may all encourage a state of mind that can optimize treatment outcome. Encouraging a sense of optimism, hope and a sense of control improves physical well-being. On the other hand, pessimism breeds passiveness and a sense of defeat experienced as 'learned helplessness'. Mind-body exercises, such as internal Qi Gong and meditation, will prime the person with cancer to heal more effectively from physical interventions, by improving the mind-body communication systems and enhancing the person's sense of control. This is often reflected by experiencing less fatigue, reduced side-effects, and an increase in the measured immune cell response.

The Main Components of Traditional ☯ Chinese Medicine

The physical interventions of Chinese Medicine include herbal therapies, acupuncture, nutrition, and massage (Tui Na). They may be utilized together or as separate treatment modalities. Also, some treatments may be generalized, such as specific patent herbal formulas for certain side-effects of radiotherapy and chemotherapy, or acupuncture treatment of specific points, such as Pericardium 6 (P6) for nausea and vomiting. However, many practitioners would add an individualized therapy plan according to TCM diagnostic criteria, that reflects the constituents of the personality and mind-body patterns. The combination of herbal therapies and nutrition to treat deficient energy, acupuncture to rebalance the energy system, and Tui Na with Qi Gong to promote continuing health, is the most powerful approach to symptom control and restoration of health.

Chinese Herbs ☯

The Chinese pharmacy is a huge compendium of pharmacologically active chemical compounds derived from plants, animal products and minerals. The preparations may be extracted from various parts of the plant or animal, and are usually mixed together into specific combinations determined by the pattern of disharmony within the information systems of a specific individual. Herbs used for the person with cancer are often categorized as *Fu zheng* and *Gu ben*. The meaning of these terms is to strengthen the person's natural healing resources, such as immunity, regeneration and repair. As such, they are useful concomitant therapies to conventional Western medicine, that focuses on tumor destruction by surgery, radiotherapy and chemotherapy. The Chinese herbs seem to counteract the toxicity imposed on normal, healthy tissues, by the side-effects of anti-cancer therapies.

❧ *Acupuncture*

Acupuncture involves the penetration of the skin by hair-like needles at specific anatomical points that may correspond to nerve pathways or receptors in tissue fascia. Different combinations of points have a wide variation of effects on symptoms, degree of inflammation, tissue regeneration, hormone levels, number of immunocytes, and the balance of the autonomic (involuntary) nervous system. The optimal selection of points requires expert knowledge and experience, and can vary between patients. In addition, the points can be tonified (stimulated) or sedated (suppressed) by appropriate patterns of physical manipulation or electrical pulsation. There are some standard acupuncture points for common symptoms, but individual patterns of disease require a unique, tailored approach.

❧ *Manipulation of Energy Flow*

Tui Na massage can be used for symptom reduction through manipulation of specific pressure points that can influence energy flow in a similar way to acupuncture. In addition, both external Qi Gong and acupuncture may involve electromagnetic information transfer from practitioner to patient that may entrain the patient's disrupted electromagnetic information flow back to a normal state. Internal Qi Gong allows the person to take control of their own energy field through a combination of appropriate exercise movements and breathing techniques. This often results in improved symptom control and less fatigue. The sensation of electrical tingling along the energy meridians during Qi Gong appears to correlate with changes in electrical potential on the skin, according to recent experiments by Dr Glen Rein, that will be referred to later in this book.

The Clinical Practice of Traditional Chinese Medicine ☯

You can expect a good practitioner of Chinese medicine to take a thorough history, concentrating on your personality type and life experience. Examination will focus on your tongue and pulse. The tongue is one of the most densely innervated organs in our body and also has a vigorous blood flow and rapid rate of epithelial cell proliferation. Changes in the balance of the autonomic nervous system, fluid balance, acid-base balance, respiration, nutrition, immunity, and many other physiological criteria will be reflected by variations in color, engorgement, thickness and geographical patterns of surface epithelium. For example, many patients having chemotherapy develop a denuded, shrunken, dry red tongue, with perhaps a scanty yellow coating, representing yin deficiency. This is partly due to restricted epithelial cell regeneration, dehydration of the tongue and inflammation. Herbs to replace yin would be appropriate. They would contain pharmacological agents to reduce inflammation, protect the membrane of the surface epithelial cells, and encourage their regeneration. Of course, the tongue is only the visible tip of the iceberg, and the herbs would be acting at other sites, such as the gastrointestinal tract, to help healing elsewhere. Therefore, gastrointestinal symptoms would be reduced, appetite increased, nutrition improved, and recovery encouraged. The pulse reflects a combination of heart beat and tone within the blood vessels, and is regulated by the autonomic nervous system. An imbalance between sympathetic and parasympathetic tone changes the pulse pattern. Since many physiological functions, including metabolism, hormone messages, immunity, blood flow and respiration, are modulated by the autonomic nervous system, the pulse pattern can be a powerful indicator of health status. The beat-to-beat variation of the heart rate also reflects sympathetic-parasympathetic balance, and is being shown scientifically to reflect a variety of health outcomes. Acupuncture, herbs and Qi Gong can all influence the balance of the autonomic nervous system and may encourage an improvement in health through harmonizing the relative contribution of the sympathetic and parasympathetic components.

☯ *Chapter Two*

The Journey to an Integrative Care Plan:
Rachel's Story

- Decision-Making

- A Holistic and Integrated Treatment Plan

- Enlightened Conventional Medicine

- Emotional Catharsis

- Supportive Care

- The Moral of the Story

☯ *Decision-Making*

Rachel is a 45 year old mother of three children who was recently diagnosed with a cancer in the left breast. She was offered a surgical excision of the lump in the breast, along with removal of lymph nodes in her axilla, followed by routine radiotherapy. Alternatively she could have had a mastectomy, but she wished to preserve her natural breast. She was anxious about having surgery and obsessed whether she had made the correct decision. Her friend suggested that she consulted with an experienced practitioner of Chinese Medicine.

☯ *A Holistic and Integrated Treatment Plan*

She was surprised that the practitioner, Dr. Susan Lo, took a very thorough history, concentrating on her daily habits and emotions, and ascertaining her reactions to the vicissitudes of life. After examining her tongue and spending some time concentrating on her pulse, she informed Rachel that she had an excess of Liver fire and a weak Spleen, and that her level of qi was low. Although the practitioner emphasized that this was not a specific cause for her cancer, she suggested that Rachel undergo some simple treatment prior to surgery in order to help with her anxiety and sleeplessness, increase her confidence in her ability to make decisions, and help her to improve her nutrition. Susan informed Rachel that the treatment would also boost her immunity, decrease surgical complications and hasten her wound healing. In addition, she suggested that Rachel obtain a ReliefBand™, an electrical device worn like a wrist watch, that electrically stimulates the P6 acupuncture point on the wrist. This would help prevent

"What is the use of a book", thought Alice,
"without pictures or conversations?"
Alice's Adventures in Wonderland by **Lewis Caroll (1865)**

nausea and vomiting following anesthesia, and would also help to reduce anxiety. Susan also suggested that she deliver several sessions of acupuncture prior to surgery, in order to reduce Rachel's agitation and anxiety, and to help her fatigue. Rachel was curious when Susan inserted the very fine needles into points in her legs and wrists. She felt a curious tingling sensation and a very mild ache in her foot, followed by a rhythmic pulsing when Susan connected the electrical stimulation to the needles. After 5 minutes, Rachel felt very relaxed and fell asleep for 20 minutes until Susan removed the needles. Following the treatment, Rachel felt calm and focused. Susan discussed some simple dietary advice, including an emphasis on a wide variety of lightly steamed vegetables, fish, and fresh fruit. In addition, she demonstrated some simple Qi Gong exercises, including one to gather qi and to cleanse the marrow. Rachel found that this maintained her calmness, and helped her to feel full of energy. Susan suggested that Rachel start taking some herbs to strengthen her qi and to reduce the excess fire in her Liver. She carefully prescribed a specific formula and wrote down the ingredients for Rachel to have available, and arranged for her physician and pharmacist to be informed. She also gave Rachel a note for her physician, to keep him informed of her plan of supportive management, and gave her contact details so that other healthcare professionals could contact her to discuss the details of the integrative care plan.

Enlightened Conventional Medicine ☯

Rachel successfully underwent surgery. Prior to the procedure, she was calm and relaxed, and suffered no complications or side-effects. Her anesthesiologist was curious about the ReliefBand™ and was remarkably surprised when it rapidly terminated her post-operative nausea and vomiting. He was compelled to do a review of the literature, in the hospital library, and was even more surprised when he discovered a series of randomized controlled trials that demonstrated the effectiveness of acupuncture stimulation of this specific point on the wrist. He wondered why such an effective procedure, with a scientific basis, and evidence-based results, was not being taught in medical schools, and was not part of routine practice.

One week later, Rachel's oncologist informed her that she had some involved lymph nodes and that she should be treated with chemotherapy to reduce the risk of recurrence from spread to other sites. In addition, he advised her that she still required radiotherapy to her breast, to prevent local recurrence. She was dismayed to hear about the side-effects of fatigue, nausea and vomiting, loss of appetite, hair loss, and early menopause. After returning home, she found relief in practicing her Qi Gong and doing some breathing exercises that her husband had taught her to do. She telephoned Susan Lo and made an appointment for the next day.

☯ *Emotional Catharsis*

Susan was very sympathetic to Rachel's fears. During their discussion, Rachel expressed a lot of anger and felt that it was unfair that she had developed cancer when she had three children to care for. Susan considered her anger to be deep-seated and had been present for a long time. She suggested that Rachel be referred for professional counseling, in order to help her resolve these issues. Meanwhile, Susan asked Rachel if she would like some energy treatment to relax her. Rachel agreed and lay down on the comfortable couch and closed her eyes. Susan proceeded to lightly touch the back of Rachel's head, her forehead, and chest, gradually working her way down to hold her feet. She waved her hands over Rachel's body and stroked the air that surrounded her. Rachel felt calm and loved. Images of crying as a baby, and having a raging tantrum as a toddler, filled her mind and then floated away, released and forgiven.

Supportive Care ☯

At the end of the session, Rachel was ready to plan her strategy for dealing with the side-effects of chemotherapy and radiotherapy. Susan suggested a patent Chinese herb formula called Chemo-Support™ to take during the chemotherapy, and a formula called Radio-Support™ for the radiotherapy (see Appendix A). In addition, she suggested weekly acupuncture to increase her energy, increase appetite, and boost her white cell count (immune cell activity). Susan planned to continue her regular Qi Gong exercises and to pay particular attention to her diet.

Rachel received long-term follow-up from her TCM practitioner as well as her oncologist. A few years later, she developed hot flashes associated with early menopause that was precipitated by the chemotherapy. Acupuncture reduced the flashes and suppressed her irritability. Susan recommended a high soy diet to help the menopausal symptoms, but thought it was wise to discuss this issue directly with Rachel's oncologist in view of some controversy regarding potential risk of precipitating recurrence through the mild estrogenic activity of soy. Rachel's oncologist did a literature search using 'Medline' on the World Wide Web, and concluded that the current evidence did not confirm an increased risk of recurrence. With a combination of acupuncture, a soy diet, and intermittent Chinese herbs, Rachel's menopause symptoms resolved.

☯ *The Moral of The Story*

Rachel's story is one of many narratives that patients have told me. Each person's story and journey is different, despite similar cancers and uniform conventional treatments. In choosing your path, it will be necessary to find out who you are as a person and as a soul. Your path is your own personal journey, during which you are not alone, but you choose your path and your companions. This will mean drawing together support from loved ones, friends, professional colleagues, spiritual counselors, and many diverse healthcare professionals. Your team may be large, but it should be focused and integrated. TCM, along with conventional practice, could be a starting point for your journey. Chinese Medicine has a lot of evaluative and therapeutic techniques to offer you. What is more, scientific research is demonstrating that it has a useful role to play in cancer treatment, side-by-side with conventional Western medicine. We start the journey together, by considering cancer from a TCM point of view, evaluating the evidence for its effectiveness, and concluding that TCM can play an important part in reducing side-effects of anti-cancer therapy, and may contribute to the potential for a sustained quality of life, and even cure. My role is to start you on this journey, to consider the scenery, and then it is up to you to decide whether you wish to travel further down this pathway. Bon voyage!

☯ *Chapter Three*

Cancer as a Systemic Disease

- Systems Theory

- The Body-Mind Network

- Communication Failure

- Chinese Herbs

- Acupuncture

☯ *Systems Theory*

In conventional Western Medicine, cancer is viewed solely from the somatic point of view as a clone of cells that has outgrown its environmental constraints and control mechanisms. These cells are abnormal and are considered to be foreign to the body. The main philosophy of cancer treatment is direct annihilation of the cancer cells using aggressive and destructive therapies. The importance of the body-mind communication network in cancer treatment has not been emphasized. In TCM, cancer is viewed as only a part of the presenting features of a syndrome representing an imbalance of the whole body-mind network[1]. In other words, cancer is a systemic disease from the start, and the terrain is considered to be as important as the tumor itself[2]. It is believed that if one can strengthen and rebalance the body-mind network, the normal pattern will be restored and this will help to resolve the cancer. Although cancer is often observed as an anatomical abnormality, it is a failure of fitness within a complex, dynamic system.

☯ *The Body-Mind Network*

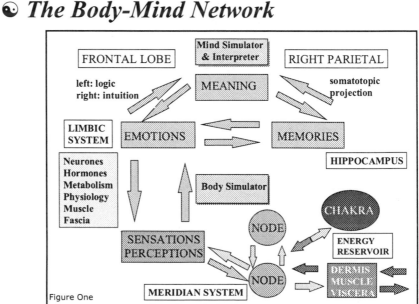

Figure One

TCM recognizes that the human being functions as a body-mind network[3] (Figure one). The philosophy of TCM analyzes the *process* of body-mind communication, rather than a 'snap shot' of structural, material entities such as molecules. If Western Medicine is viewed as the hardware of a computer, then TCM would be seen as the software. It recognizes a correspondence between patterns of information that are independent of the carrier of the information. For example, the pattern of information may be similar regardless of whether it is mediated by pulses of hormones and neuropeptides, or the electrophysiological frequency pattern of the heart[4-8]. Acupuncture stimulation of specific points on the body releases neuropeptides (such as somatostatin and vasoactive intestinal peptide) within the central nervous system[9-10]. The body-mind information system may be partly regulated by the relative contributions of the sympathetic and parasympathetic components of the autonomic nervous system. This corresponds to the traditional Chinese concept of a balance between yin and yang, that represents a pattern of information, rather than concrete material entities. Analysis of the pulse, using the classical Chinese technique, may indicate the relative imbalance. This has been demonstrated indirectly by spectral analysis of the electrocardiogram, using appropriate computer software. My research colleagues are currently developing a system to analyze the pulse wave spectrum directly, using a transducer and a computerized analysis. Acupuncture has been shown to rebalance the relative contributions of the sympathetic and parasympathetic nervous systems[11]. The patterns of information transfer may interact to entrain and reinforce information flow in a complex dynamical system[12-14]. The system is an autopoietic process, that is it can recreate itself and evolve through learning, so that the body can adapt to changing circumstances.

> When something grows, something else will decay. When something disappears, something else emerges. This is the balance of things. If there is only growth and no decay, the world will be overpopulated, be it with people, animals, or vegetation. If there is only decay and no growth, life will disappear. For the world to continue there must be a balance of growth and decay.
> *Taoist hermit Lieh Tzu, (born 400 BCE)*

☯ *Communication Failure*

When we are healthy, communication between systems flows freely in a complex, non-linear heterarchical and hierarchical process of information flow. Cancer may be associated with a disturbance in information flow, manifest by an over-plastic system that loses process structure and becomes irreversibly chaotic[15-16]. Intervention with a technique, such as acupuncture, may restore the imbalance in information flow, for example through the autonomic nervous system by balancing the sympathetic and parasympathetic components[17-18]. The same model may help us understand how the compassionate intentionality of a healer can restore health through entrainment and normalization of the imbalanced system[19]. In order to understand these processes, we will need to consider systems outside of our current reductionist, pharmacological model. These may include electromagnetic and non-local effects between molecules, and the analysis of information flow between cells by quantum mechanics[20]. In order to understand the concurrent, synergistic contributions of multiple systems, it is necessary to develop computerized algorithmic modeling, such as power spectral analysis[11], neural networks[21], and fuzzy logic[22] (modern techniques used for processing information).

The beauty of this body-mind network model is that it can combine constitutional personality factors (such as emotions and feelings) with bodily symptoms, into a single diagnostic and treatment paradigm. This is represented in TCM terms by patterns of disharmonies in the main Organ systems, as well as abnormalities of qi (energy flow), essence (energy reserves), blood (energy supply), heat (energy expenditure) and moisture (fluid balance). It is interesting that there is correspondence with the

TCM model of cancer predisposition. Cancer is associated with rising qi (sheng qi) or liver fire (representing anger). Recent scientific evidence suggests that repressed anger both suppresses the immune system, and may increase the risk of breast cancer in the so-called Type C personality [23-25].

Chinese Herbs ☯

In TCM, herbs are used in combinations that enhance their benefits while reducing their side-effects[26]. In effect, multiple low dose pharmaceutical agents are being administered synergistically. This is in complete contrast to our Western model that focuses on a high dose effect of a single pharmaceutical agent. The interaction of low doses of pharmacologically active agents with the wide spectrum of both homologous and heterogeneous cell membrane receptors, may enable a more gradual shift in cell function, with minimal adverse side-effects and less tolerance to the active agents. A skilled Chinese pharmacist is very necessary in order to prepare the correct balance of herbs. The administration of single agents at high dose will simply induce many of the disadvantages of conventional pharmaceutical agents, such as severe side-effects, tolerance, and addiction. Moreover, an appropriate shift in the *natural* pattern of interaction between local hormones, neurotransmitters, and intracellular signaling chemicals is more likely to enable a *natural* shift back to the normal health-orientated homeostatic state. The administration of herbs without the advice of a certified TCM practitioner cannot be condoned in view of the complexity of mixing appropriate herbs in the correct proportions, and being aware that inappropriate combinations or doses can result in possibly serious side-effects. Moreover, the model for administration of the herbs is not based on conventional pharmacology,

> Better is a dinner of herbs where love is, than a stalled ox and hatred therewith.
> *Old Testament: Proverbs xv. 17.*

> You don't get harmony when everybody sings the same note.
> *Doug Floyd*

but on an energetic model that considers imbalances in corresponding levels of information flow. This is often diagnosed at the level of the whole person (such as emotional balance). However, it is related to imbalances of chemicals at the cellular level. Some herbs are available 'ready-mixed' and are termed patent preparations, for example Chemo-Support™ (see Appendix A), that reduces symptoms of chemotherapy treatment. This is a carefully prepared and quality-assured product that maintains an accurate combination of herbs. However, the seasoned practitioner will often add in other herbs to individualize the prescription according to constitutional and personality attributes.

In summary, harmony is restored through the complex pattern of herbal chemicals interacting with the dynamic information flow of molecules within and between cells. This system encompasses much more than conventional pharmacology, and is called energetics. Energetic harmony is ultimately a field effect, incorporating all body-mind functions, and may be envisioned, and possibly measured, by detecting changes in electromagnetic energy flow.

☯ *Acupuncture*

Most evidence suggests that acupuncture modulates neurotransmitters, cytokines and neuropeptides through electrophysiological changes in the nervous system[27-28]. Interaction with the brain stem, hypothalamus, limbic system and autonomic nervous system occurs through either stimulating or suppressing the activity of afferent peripheral nerves[29-34]. Acupuncture may also modify the somatic electromagnetic field[35]. It is a technique that allows us to modulate communication within the body-mind network through concurrent changes in multiple signaling pathways. Similar to the use of herbs, the use of acupuncture within the context of Chinese Medicine is to restore harmony of information flow, that is reflected by energetic field theory. Metaphorically, it modulates information flow like an orchestral conductor, directing the individual instruments and their wide spectrum of musical notes into a coordinated harmony. Acupuncture may be used to redirect energy (information and capacity to do work) at various physiological levels. However, in some patients who are very weak in qi (ability to do work by having adequate energy flow) herbs are often a pre-requisite before acupuncture is used to redirect the energy flow and restore the harmony of health.

Like everything else in nature, music is a becoming, and it becomes its full self, when its sounds and laws are used by intelligent man for the production of harmony, and so made the vehicle of emotion and thought.
Theodore Mungers

☯ *Chapter Four*

Integration of Traditional Chinese Medicine into Cancer Supportive Care

- Goals of Cancer Treatment

- More Questions than Answers

- Alchemy

- The Mystical Oncologist

- The Mystery and Science of Traditional Chinese Medicine

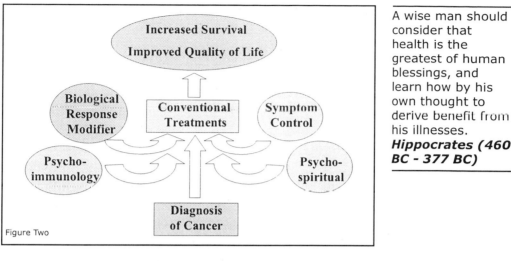

Figure Two

A wise man should consider that health is the greatest of human blessings, and learn how by his own thought to derive benefit from his illnesses.
Hippocrates (460 BC - 377 BC)

Goals of Cancer Treatment ☯

The goals of cancer treatment should be to increase survival, when possible, and to improve quality of life. TCM is able to support patients being treated with conventional Western Medicine (surgery, radiotherapy and chemotherapy) through four major approaches:

(1) Biological response modification;
(2) Improvement of psycho-neuro-immunological function;
(3) Improvement of symptom control;
(4) Improvement of psycho-spiritual well being.

Very often, TCM therapy works through more than one approach, synergistically (Figure two).

We should manage our fortunes as we do our health - enjoy it when good, be patient when it is bad, and never apply violent remedies except in an extreme necessity.
Francois de La Rochefoucauld (1613-1680)

More Questions than Answers ☯

Can we integrate conventional medicine with an ancient traditional healthcare system, based on intuitive philosophy and many years of observing the behavior and response of individuals (rather than populations) to non-technological

If the facts don't fit the theory, change the facts.
Albert Einstein (1879-1955)

interventions? Is three thousand years of 'enlightened' observation equivalent to one randomized controlled trial or, indeed, a meta-analysis? Is the cultural background of TCM relevant to North American Society? Do we need an alternative healthcare system?

These are all important questions and there is a lot of validity in taking a critical approach. Inappropriate interventions may delay the use of proven therapies. Toxicity can occur from adverse combinations of chemotherapy and some herbs. The quality assurance and content of many herbal products is uncertain. False hope, unnecessary expenditure, guilt, and burn-out from information-seeking, are all potential risks when embarking down a pathway of integrating alternative therapies with conventional care.

I believe that we can integrate the best of both healthcare systems, so long as we do it in a structured, ethical, quality-assured, and evidence-based manner. We need to be intelligent. Scientific evaluation *is* still possible within the context of a humanistic, individual and relationship-centered care plan. The essential skill is to balance the science of objectivity and abstraction with the metaphysics of individual subjectivity.

☯ *Alchemy*

Scientific methodology should not be confused with the mystery and magic of relationship-centered care. In addition, we need explanations of efficacy in terms of both molecular interactions and metaphorical metaphysics. People do not usually identify themselves with collections of interacting molecules, but they often see themselves as individual spirits and distinct colorful entities. People identify themselves within the context of their families. Rarely do they see themselves as abstractions of population surveys. Yet, unfortunately, scientific data is often presented in an unreal context, stripped of its personality, meaning, and emotions, reduced to a skeleton of objectivity, torn from the subjective feelings and individuality that made the data relevant to the human state of being. A re-introduction of alchemy into medicine is long overdue. The practice of medicine is *not* science. It *is* an amalgam of generalized scientific data, based on current theories, integrated with the art of healing the individual patient. It should be a mixture of technology and ancient human-based healing skills. As we scientifically investigate the ability of humans to heal each other, we are finding fascinating ways in which this healing information can be transferred. Our ultimate power as healers is to appropriately synthesize a rapprochement of technology-based interventions with the traditional approaches of ancient wisdom.

The Mystical Oncologist ☯

In my own practice, I am comfortable talking in terms of molecules, enzyme activities, genetics, and chemical reactions, as well as chakras (energy centers), acupoints, vital spirit, etheric and astral energy levels, in addition to other scientific and esoteric metaphysical realms. I fine tune my language according to my patients' sensitivities, deep personal beliefs, and cultural background. I never force my opinions, but guide them to places within themselves, where they can explore their own core values, meaning and purpose. In a safe and healing environment, they can explore their own deep mysteries, faith, and intuitive beliefs. Then I will bring them back from the metaphysical world and into the realms of objectivity, statistical data, population studies, and best scientific evidence. We may then travel full circle, back into the dimensions of mystery, hope, creativity, longing, and ultimately peace. I walk in their moccasins and they can walk in mine. We are in this journey together, as travelling companions. The journey for exploring a therapeutic plan is a lot longer and more arduous than a simple decision board or flow chart. It must take into account the complexities of being human.

☯ *The Mystery and Science of Traditional Chinese Medicine*

Traditional Chinese Medicine incorporates the constitutional complexities of being human. It synthesizes the relationship of the intangible elements of the human personality and experience with environmental influences. It formulates a treatment plan based on the individual person's experience. It evaluates in terms of *process* and *function,* rather than anatomical entities. However, this does not preclude measuring the efficacy of TCM interventions. Observation and record-keeping have been traditionally cherished within the Chinese culture. It is only recently that many of these texts have been translated into the English language. Even then, the true richness of meaning is often lost, since it is difficult to accurately convey the original understanding into terms we appreciate today. Ironically, much of the meaning and comprehension is understood better within the terminology of quantum physics, rather than our current conservative medical terminology. Despite these challenges, studies of TCM interventions are being published, some in reputable conventional medical journals. This research needs to continue and an evidence-based collage of TCM is gradually forming. We still have no specific definition for qi, and we still do not fully understand why mixtures of many herbs should have advantages over highly refined pharmaceuticals. Does Qi Gong heal? Does acupuncture really work, or is it just a placebo effect? Which acupuncture points work for which conditions? Why do we need different patterns of acupoints for the same symptoms in different people? Read on, and perhaps you too will be enlightened!

☯ *Chapter Five*

Biological Response Modification: A Balance of Yin and Yang

- Adjuvant Therapy and Therapeutic Gain

- Complementary Herbs

- Modulation of Tumor Response by Electro-acupuncture

Adjuvant Therapy and Therapeutic Gain ☯

Traditional Chinese Medicine can be added to conventional cancer treatments, such as chemotherapy, radiotherapy, and surgery, in order to facilitate the therapeutic effect of the conventional therapy. We can potentially increase the therapeutic gain, that is, enhance the cancer-killing activity *plus* reduce toxic side-effects. The current understanding of molecular biology suggests that both herbs and acupuncture influence the local communicating hormones that transmit messages between cells. Therefore, selective herbs and specific combinations of acupuncture points can modify an imbalance of these molecules, that in turn can increase the kill of cancer cells and reduce the side-effects on normal tissue. Some of these communicating molecules include the cytokines, that are proteins released by our immune cells to kill foreign invading cells and to attract more cancer-fighting cells. Others include derivatives of fatty acids, such as the prostaglandins, that balance inflammatory effects, such as blood flow and leakage of intravascular fluid into the tissues.

In obtaining therapeutic gain and optimizing the death of cancer cells, whilst minimizing damage to our own functioning cells and tissues, it is important to buffer the toxic effects of chemotherapy and surgery. A specific example is the toxic effect of the spread of free radicals induced by radiation therapy and some chemotherapy agents. Free radicals are very reactive species of oxygen that can cause major damage to the chains of nucleic acids that form our genetic material, as well as destruction of cell membranes. These free radicals cause long-term damage to our tissues, and suppression of our immunological defense system. Consequently, agents that can allow the free radicals to poison cancer cells whilst sparing normal tissue

Strength should always be complemented by softness. If you resist too much, you will break. Thus, the strong person knows when to use strength and when to yield, and good fortune and disaster depend on whether you know how and when to yield.
Taoist hermit Lieh Tzu, (born 400 BCE)

cells can increase the therapeutic gain. Some Chinese herbs are antioxidants that can mop-up an excess of free radicals, allowing them to destroy cancer cells, but terminating their activity before they can damage non-cancer tissue. In Chinese terminology, yang is allowed to attack the cancer cells, but is balanced by yin that restores and sustains an environment suitable for our normal tissue cells to quickly recover.

There is increasing evidence that suggests that TCM can favorably modify the tumor response to conventional Western cancer treatment. There are correspondences between the TCM theory of cancer and recent medical research findings.

❧ *Complementary Herbs*

TCM herbs have been extensively investigated in the laboratory and are known to have multiple pharmacological effects [36-41]. It is often important to specify the botanical parts from which the herbal agent is prepared, since the active pharmacological agents depend on their source. Radix (Rx) denotes the root, Cortex (Cx) denotes the bark or rind, and Rhizome (Rh) denotes the rhizome. *Rx Ginseng* has anti-tumor activity, inhibits platelet aggregation, and inhibits chemotherapy-induced immunosuppression. *Glycyrrhizic acid* has anti-tumor activity, is anti-inflammatory through increasing serum cortisol, and also increases natural killer (NK) cell activity against cancer cells. *Rx Astragali membranaceus* is a powerful stimulator of the immune system, has anti-tumor activity and inhibits platelet aggregation. *Rx Angelica sinensis* stimulates the immune system, has anti-tumor activity, inhibits platelet aggregation, and inhibits vascular permeability. *Rh Atractylodis macrocephala* has anti-tumor activity, and is an anti-thrombotic and fibrinolytic agent. *Ginkgo biloba* has multiple effects including inhibition of platelet activation factor (PAF), stimulation of the immune system, fibrinolyis and anti-thrombosis activity, scavenging of free radicals, and dilation of blood vessels to increase perfusion.

These herbs contain a variety of chemicals that may act synergistically to inhibit tumor cell division, increase tumor cell death (apoptosis), increase the proportion of immune cells within the tumor, and increase blood flow through the tumor. This is associated with a change in the balance of cytokines (communicating peptides released by the immune cells) that may improve the *therapeutic gain*. This means that they reduce the proliferation of tumor cells, increase tumor cell death, whilst minimizing many side-effects for normal tissues. Examples of studies that illustrate these principles will be discussed.

In TCM, the malignant tumor is viewed as being associated with stagnation of qi (energy) and blood. Qi may be viewed as a model for intra- and inter-cellular information and potential energy transfer. This would correlate with the known abnormalities of signal transduction, cell contact, and electrophysiology of cancer cells[15,16,41]. It has been shown that there is increased fluid content and a stagnant blood supply in a malignant tumor[42-45]. The microcirculation within a tumor is very abnormal, and there are regions within the tumor where the blood flow is sluggish. In TCM, stagnation of blood is classically associated with tumors. The impaired blood circulation leads to areas of poor oxygenation in the tumor. Cancer cells that survive in a low oxygen tension environment are also found to be more resistant to radiotherapy and some types of chemotherapy[46-47].

In TCM, destagnation or detoxification herbs are used to move the blood and qi within the malignant tumor so as to 'soften and disperse' it. Interestingly, the use of anticoagulants, such as heparin and warfarin (coumadin), as an adjunctive treatment to chemotherapy, has been shown to prevent the development of blood-borne metastases in animal laboratory studies, and to improve the survival of cancer patients in clinical studies[48-49].

The possible usefulness of *destagnation herbs* was demonstrated in a randomized controlled clinical trial evaluating the combined modality treatment of Chinese herbal destagnation formula and radiotherapy in patients with nasopharyngeal carcinoma[50]. In this trial, 90 patients received combined herbal and radiation treatment compared to 98 patients who were randomized to receive radiation treatment alone. The ingredients of the herbal formula included *Rx Astragali membranaceus, Rx Paeoniae rubrae, Rx Ligustici Chuan xiong, Rx Angelicae sinensis, Semen persica, Flos Carthami tinctorii, Rx et Caulis Jixueteng, Rx Puerariae, Pericarpium citri reticulatae*, and *Rx Codonopsitis pilosulae*. The combined treatment group showed a statistically significant increase in local tumor control and overall five-year survival as compared with the group treated with radiation alone. The rate of local recurrence in the intervention group was halved from 29% in those receiving radiation alone, to 14% in the group receiving destagnation herbs as well. The 5-year disease-free survival was increased from 37% in the control group to 53% in the group receiving destagnation herbs. It is postulated that this herbal destagnation formula may have improved tumor microcirculation and increased tumor blood flow, leading to an improvement in the oxygen tension inside the tumor. The oxygen tension increases the radiosensitivity of the tumor. In other words, the destagnation formula has acted as a radiation sensitizer.

In animal experiments, *Ginkgo biloba* has also been shown to increase perfusion and radiosensitivity[51-52].

Chinese herbs, such as *Salviae miltiorrhizae*, that inhibit tumor edema caused by free radicals may also increase tumor perfusion, oxygenation and response to radiotherapy[53-54]. Other herbs may directly sensitize neoplastic cells to radiotherapy[55]. More clinical trials should be done to further evaluate this promising role of herbs, and tumor blood flow monitored using non-invasive techniques such as functional MRI and positron emission tomography[45].

Modulation of Tumor Response by ☯ *Electro-acupuncture*

The interaction of acupuncture with appropriate acupoints modulates blood flow[17,18,56-57]. This may be through a local effect via release of cytokines, or through neurological reflexes that adjust the balance between the sympathetic and parasympathetic nervous system. Its effect on tumor physiology and response to therapy remains to be investigated. However, we do know that electric pulses to the tumor can increase the response to chemotherapy. A phase II study of electrochemotherapy using cisplatin in patients with skin nodules from malignant melanoma demonstrated a significantly increased control rate compared to cisplatin alone[58].

☯ *Chapter Six*

Enhancement of Immunity

- The Immune System and Tumor Growth

- Immune Deficiency

- Inoculations, Coley's Toxins and Other Immuno-therapies

- Terrain versus the Seed: The Immune-Enhancing Herbs

- Terrain versus the Seed: Manipulation of the Immune Response with Acupuncture

- The Hormone Balancing Act

The Immune System and Tumor Growth ☯

Can the immune system regulate the growth of cancers? We talk about the immune system surveying the body and fighting cancer cells. Is this speculation or does it really occur? According to Burnet's immune surveillance theory, cells that express surface proteins that are recognized as 'foreign' are destroyed by specific immune cells. These are usually thymus-derived lymphocytes, so-called T cells, and natural killer cells, so-called NK cells. These cells will often go on a 'suicide' mission to destroy a cancer cell by releasing toxic enzymes and reactive oxygen species (free radicals) in the vicinity of the renegade cell. However, in addition to this dramatic attack, there are many other more subtle ways that the immune system can control cancer cells. The immunocytes are constantly releasing communication molecules, such as cytokines, that are often small protein messenger molecules which can attract (or repel) other cells, influence them to divide (or to remain dormant), and modulate the chemical reactions within the other cells. Other chemicals, derived from fatty acids and called prostaglandins, may be involved. The activity of the immune cells is intricately connected to the endocrine system that produces messenger molecules called hormones. There is also interaction with the nervous system, and this will be discussed in the next chapter.

> "Illnesses hover constantly above us, their seeds blown by the wind, but they do not set in the terrain unless the terrain is ready to receive them."
> **Claude Bernard (1813-1878)**

Immune Deficiency ☯

We know that suppression of immunity by certain drugs (specifically those used in preventing organ transplant rejection) results in an increased risk of many cancers. In addition, the Acquired Immunodeficiency Disease Syndrome (AIDS), such as that caused by the Human

Immunodeficiency Virus (HIV), is associated with cancers such as lymphomas and a rare skin tumor called Kaposi sarcoma. The development of cervix (womb) cancer is associated both with an infection by the Human Papilloma Virus and suppression of the immune cells in the cervix by smoking cigarettes. Yes, the toxins from smoking can penetrate further than the lungs! Some of these tumors can remit when the immune cell count recovers. In addition, immune-enhancing therapies with the communicating proteins released by immunocytes (cytokines, such as interferon and the interleukins) can produce limited anti-tumor responses when used to treat malignant melanoma (an aggressive skin cancer) and kidney cancer. However, the doses used in therapy are far above the levels found in normal cell-to-cell communication, and the mechanisms of cancer cell destruction are still unclear.

❧ *Inoculations, Coley's Toxins and other Immuno-therapies*

Animal models suggest that the anti-tumor cytotoxicity (that is the cell-killing ability) of the NK lymphocytes, and the localized inflammatory response mediated by CD4 lymphocytes (so-called helper cells), can influence tumor growth and metastasis. However, few studies have been done on human beings to determine whether a similar mechanism occurs. What we do know is that immune cells from humans can be sensitized to attack cancer cells, by removing them from the person with cancer, exposing them to the foreign protein found on the cancer cells, giving them a 'boost of energy' by stimulating them with cytokines (such as the interleukins) and then re-injecting them back into the host. This therapy is similar to inoculation, vaccination or 'having a shot'. Less specific ways of enhancing the immune response include the injection of inactivated bacteria. The surface wall of the bacteria contains components (lipopolysaccharides) that stimulate immune cell activity, release of cancer-killing chemicals, and fever. One of these toxic chemicals is appropriately called Tumor Necrosis Factor (TNF). The body's natural response to the injection of lipopolysaccharides is toxic to cancer cells. This type of therapy was initially pioneered by a famous surgeon called William Coley, the father of immunotherapy. Research on his approach continues. However, another type of inoculation called BCG, that is usually used as a 'shot' against tuberculosis (TB), is effective in stimulating an immune response that can suppress early bladder cancer.

There is enough preliminary evidence to suggest that the immune system plays a vital role in the defense against cancer progression. TCM uses a combination of techniques to enhance the immune response, including herbs, acupuncture, and Qi Gong.

Terrain versus the Seed: ☯
The Immune-Enhancing Herbs

Another strategy that TCM uses in cancer therapy is to strengthen the whole body-mind system by enhancing and harmonizing the energy balance between all the Organs. This may be viewed as correcting an imbalance in the body-mind communication network and is reflected by an enhancement in immunity. This is called *Fu Zheng* treatment and is mediated by the specific group of TCM herbs called *Fu Zheng* herbs[59-70]. There is evidence that improvement of the immunological function of cancer patients is associated with an improvement in their survival. In China, *Fu Zheng* herbs have been reported to increase survival when combined with radiotherapy for patients with nasopharyngeal cancer, and when combined with chemotherapy for patients with stomach and liver cancer[1,71].

Fu Zheng herbs, including *Rx Ginseng, Ganoderma, Rx Astragali membranaceus, Rx Angelicae sinensis, Cordyceps sinensis and Fructus Lycii*, have been shown to enhance the body's defense mechanisms. Clinical studies, including two randomized trials, have found that the NK cell and OKT4 (immune-enhancing lymphocyte) cell counts were increased with the use of *Fu Zheng* herbs[59-70]. These immunocytes are known to attack cancer cells. In a study of gastric cancer patients, increased survival was found in the combined treatment group, receiving both *Fu Zheng* herbs and chemotherapy, versus the chemotherapy alone group. Many of these herbs are associated with an increase in cytokines, such as interferon and interleukin[72-74]. Chinese studies also suggest that healing of normal tissues may be enhanced. Anti-inflammatory constituents may diminish radiation-induced ulcers and chemotherapy-induced stomatitis [75-76].

☯ *Terrain versus the Seed: Manipulation of the Immune Response with Acupuncture*

Multiple animal and clinical studies have also suggested that acupuncture has a positive immune-modulating effect in cancer patients[77-86]. In these studies, acupuncture has been shown to increase T-lymphocyte proliferation, increase NK cell activities, activate the complement system and heat-stable mitogenic humoral factor, and increase OKT4 cell counts. Inhibition of the growth of transplanted mammary cancer has also been shown in mice with the use of acupuncture. The main acupoints that were used in these studies were those that support blood formation and Spleen function. These points include LI 4, LI 11, St 36,

Sp 6, Sp10, P6, UB 20, GB39 and GV14. An increased level of all components (red blood cells, white blood cells and platelets) was found.

The Hormone Balancing Act ☯

Some Chinese herbs inhibit hormone-responsive tumor cells. PC-SPES is a combination of herbs with estrogenic effects, associated with activity against prostate cancer[87]. This study, which was published in the New England Journal of Medicine (a prestigious mainstream medical journal), correlated laboratory activity with clinical response. Acupuncture may stimulate steroid levels and other hormones, such as melatonin, somatostatin, and vasoactive intestinal peptide (VIP), that could potentially have anti-tumor effects[9-10, 88]. The exposure to bright light of a location behind the knee, over which runs the Bladder meridian, modulates the circadian release of melatonin from the pineal gland[89]. We know that acupuncture points can be stimulated by light, and that acupuncture therapy can be administered using light from a low energy laser source.

Combinations of herbs and acupuncture can change the balance between the different types of immune cells and the pattern of hormone levels. In many situations, this subtle change will influence tumor control only when they are used with powerful conventional therapies, such as chemotherapy and radiation. In some rare situations, dramatic tumor responses can be seen when changing the ambient terrain. The problem is that we currently have no reliable way of predicting the responders. The response may depend on many variables in tumor cell receptor levels, sensitivity to immune cell attacks, and responsiveness to growth control inhibition by various agents of negative feedback. Until we have better data, the use of immune cell enhancement and endocrine (hormone) manipulation should usually be implemented as an adjuvant to proven conventional therapies. Rarely, when there is appropriate published data, a TCM herbal combination may be used as an alternative. An example is PC-SPES that is sometimes used for metastatic or advanced prostate cancer, and is known to have anti-androgen activity.

☯ *Chapter Seven*

Psychoneuroimmunology

- Descartes is Dead

- Modern Psycho-Neuro-Immunology:
  The State of the Art

- The Yellow Emperor's Version of Psycho-
  Neuro-Immunology

- Who am I?

- The Embodied Mind

- The Autonomic Nervous System: A
  Balance of Yin and Yang

- The Heart of the Matter: Compassion and
  Electromagnetic Field Effects

- Possibilities, Probabilities and Divination:
  Genetic Expression and the I Ching

- Dynamical Systems and
  Energy-Information Transfer

- Disrupted Harmony: Chaos and Cancer

- Psychological Repression and
  Physical Expression

- Psychological attitude, Stress, Depression
  and Clinical Outcome

- Treatment of Depression with TCM

☯ *Descartes is Dead*

Psychoneuroimmunology (PNI) is a scientific discipline that has provided evidence of a dynamic mutual interaction between the mind, nervous system, endocrine system, and immunity. The interaction of emotions and immunocytes through molecules, such as neuropeptides, is now well-recognized. In fact, the immune system can be viewed as a complex evolutionary communication system within the body-mind network[4,115-118]. TCM recognizes this complex interaction between personality, mood states, and susceptibility to illness through malfunction of the body-mind network.

Current scientific evidence has shown that there is communication between neurons and the immune system through so-called neural networks and a dynamic circulation of immunocytes. We now know that there is an intimate, dynamic relationship between cognition, emotions, and the functional integrity of the immune system. The renowned pathologist, David Felton first discovered that the spleen contains nerve fibers that are intimately associated with the cells of the immune system, such as lymphocytes, plasma cells, macrophages, and natural killer cells. Moreover, both the nerve endings *and* the immune cells produce similar message molecules, such as the neuropeptides, well described by Candace Pert as the "molecules of emotion". The bone marrow was also found to contain these nerve endings. Many of the neurons originate in the brain stem (or reptilian brain), especially from a site called the locus coeruleus. This site is especially significant because it, in turn, interacts with the whole brain through a sophisticated neural net, that can selectively activate locations responsible for different functions. Another major pathway connecting the immune cells to the brain is via the large vagus nerve that innervates

---

Our emotions are the result of our beliefs.
(Taoist hermit Lieh Tzu, born 400 BCE)

...The Way cannot be grasped with your senses and thoughts. Look for it in front and it will sneak behind you. Seek it with good intentions and it is everywhere. If you are insincere, it will never reveal itself. It is something that you cannot use your intellect to attain, but if you are not serious, it will also escape you. Only in naturalness can the way be attained. And after you have attained it, only in naturalness can it be kept.
(Taoist hermit Lieh Tzu, born 400 BCE)

---

the abdominal structures, including the gastrointestinal tract. Work done by John Bienenstock at McMaster University, Hamilton revealed the subtle association between immunocytes and the plexus of neurons that form, metaphorically, a gastrointestinal brain. Immune cells are formed in the thymus gland (in front of the heart), the spleen (and bone marrow) and the gastrointestinal tract. The current scientific evidence suggests a communication system that is analogous to the Organ systems described by TCM.

> Express yourself completely,
> then keep quiet.
> Be like the forces of nature:
> When it blows, there is only wind;
> When it rains, there is only rain;
> When the clouds pass, the sun shines through.
> **Tao Te Ching**

Modern Psycho-Neuro- Immunology: ☯ The State of the Art

What do we know about the function of this intricate network? Work done by Esther Sternberg at the National Institute of health showed that peptides involved in attracting immune cells are actually released by neurons in the brain, as well as by nerve endings and immunocytes. Examples include interleukin-1 and interleukin-6 (Il-1, Il-6) and tumor necrosis factor (TNF). A hormone called corticotrophin releasing factor (CRF) is also found in the brain and appears to play a powerful role in setting the level of immunity in early life, and is heavily influenced by stressful childhood experiences. High levels of CRF increase the release of adrenocortical trophic hormone (ACTH) from the pituitary gland at the base of the brain, and this stimulates the adrenal glands, that are located in the abdomen (just above the kidneys) to secrete increased levels of corticosteroids, that suppress the function of the immune cells. There is also a negative feedback loop from the immune cells back to the brain via the vagus nerve, through the secretion of Il-1, Il-6, and TNF. Immune activity can also be suppressed by the secretion of norepinephrine from the nerve endings that innervate the spleen and bone marrow. There is clearly an underlying scientific reason how emotions can effect our immunity and predispose us to certain illnesses such as cancer. There is increasing evidence that stress early in life can predispose us to serious illness as an adult. In a paper published in the prestigious medical journal, the Lancet *(1995; 346: p104)*, Licinio describes how CRF hormone binds widely to the surface receptors of cells in the body and activates an intracellular signaling (or message) system that generates the product of a gene called pro-opiomelanocortin promoter (POMC). Elements of POMC are also contained in some cancer-promoting genes, called oncogenes, such as c-fes and MAT-1, that are known to promote neoplastic transformation, that is they can cause cancer.

☯ *The Yellow Emperor's Version of Psycho-Neuro-Immunology*

The depletion of Kidney essence and jing is well described in TCM theory. Excess production of CRF hormone during early life and onwards depletes our Kidney essence and jing. Psycho-immunological burn-out is now recognized in conventional medicine. The system of TCM provides interventions to prevent the detrimental effects of stress. These therapies include nutrition, exercise and Qi Gong, herbal supplements to restore essence and qi, as well as acupuncture to channel qi and restore harmony in an imbalanced system. We can now view this restoration of birth essence and boosting of qi as a restoration of balance between the various molecules that dynamically communicate between the emotional mind and the immunological mind. Both types of mind have an enormous influence on both our psychological and physical well-being. Moreover, we are beginning to understand how an imbalance in cell-to-cell communication can allow the proliferation of neoplastic cells and the development of cancer.

Who Am I? ☯

During fetal development, cells are recognized as being part of the self by the evolving immune system. Specifically, it recognizes self through proteins on the cell membrane called major histocompatiblity antigens (MHA's). Subsequently, foreign cells are recognized as non-self because they carry different MHA's on their surface. Dendritic cells present these foreign proteins to lymphocytes, that can subsequently mount a complex attack system against the perceived invaders. Part of the defense against cancer cells may be through the recognition of abnormal, mutated MHA's that are recognized by our immune cells as not belonging to self. Some cancers carry tumor-specific antigens that are clearly foreign to self. Unfortunately, many cancer cells are crafty, and can present MHA's that are the same as normal tissues, thus providing a passport to escape part of the defense system. There is a complex modulating system that attempts to maintain the immune system under control, providing a balance between deficient immunity and an exaggerated immune response that can damage normal tissues. We are discovering increasing links with the nervous system, suggesting that states of mind and emotions can influence the subtle control mechanisms of our immune defense system. For example, the lateral hypothalamus (part of the emotional brain or limbic system) can influence the delayed hypersensitivity skin test reactivity and the natural killer cell levels in the blood. The same locus in the brain is associated with the emotions of fear and anxiety. We experience fear and anxiety in the gut, confirming the link between our cranial brain and the gastrointestinal brain, one of the major organ brains. The dorsomedial nucleus and basal ganglia of the thalamus (major junctions between the cerebral brain, emotional brain, reptilian brain, and the organ brains) relate emotional feelings to sensory information and movement. The periaqueductal grey matter (PAGM) in the brain stem, or reptilian brain, can influence functions of lymphocytes and natural killer cells. Recent studies of brain function have demonstrated that acupuncture influences activity in the PAGM. The imaging techniques of positron emission tomography (PET) and functional MRI (fMRI) produce beautiful pictures of changes in blood flow in the brain stem and thalamus, that we now know can influence our immune cell response. Even more interesting, is that the left cerebral hemisphere (the more reductionist and logical brain) and the right cerebral hemisphere (the more holistic and artistic brain) differ in their ability to influence immune cells, such as lymphocytes. Details and scientific references are well described by Bruce Rabin MD in his book, "Stress Immune Function and Health", as well as the eloquent book by Esther M. Sternberg MD, called, "The Balance Within: The Science Connecting Health and Emotions" (see Appendix B).

☯ *The Embodied Mind*

As we have ascertained from TCM theory, there is no separation between the mind and body, and it would appear that any experience is part of a system whose mind is not confined to the central nervous system, but is widely distributed throughout the body where it can influence the function of organs and the immune system. At the level of conscious awareness, we can influence this system indirectly through states of mind, metaphors and images. In addition, the system can be influenced by musculo-skeletal positioning, through kinesthetic postures and gymnastics, and acupressure points. These body information processing systems feed back to the central nervous system through proprioceptors (that sense position) and so-called afferent peripheral nerves. Therefore, the TCM philosophy of combining exercises of posture, movement, and mental imaging may have a rational scientific reason for improving health outcome.

The Autonomic Nervous System: ☯
A Balance of Yin and Yang

The autonomic nervous system (ANS) appears to play a major role as conductor of the orchestra that forms the mind-body system. Harmony between the various instruments, such as balance of immune cells, intracellular messaging systems, regulation of cell division, and metabolic activity are influenced by balance between the sympathetic and parasympathetic components of the nervous system. This is reflected by the heart rate variability (HRV), that is the beat-to-beat variation of the heart. A reduced HRV is associated with increased sympathetic and decreased parasympathetic activity (Figure three).

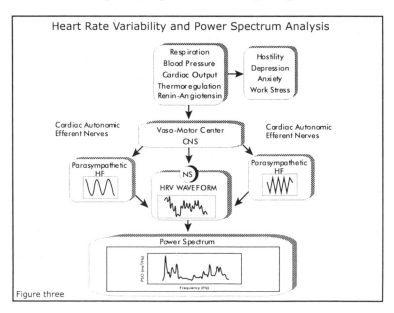

Figure three

In TCM terminology, the heart is key to a balance between loss of soul (or major depression) and excessive joy (mania, lack of focus, and exhaustion). Indeed, the heart is the seat of the spirit or mind, termed the shen. The heart appears to influence our brain waves and our states of mind. Indeed, there appears to be a mutual interaction between the electromagnetic field of the heart and the ANS via feedback to the brain[8]. We now know that decreased HRV is associated with both depression and reduced immune function. In a large epidemiological survey (the Zutphen Study) low HRV was associated with a 50% increase in the relative risk of death, including cancer. Gann and colleagues published a study that evaluated the associated risk of prostate cancer with HRV (*Cancer Epidemiol, Biomarkers, Prevention 1995; 4: 611*) and found a 1.26 relative risk when the heart rate was 10 beats per minute higher. They speculated that local trophic messenger molecules (such as neural and epithelial growth factors) were released at higher levels within the prostate gland when sympathetic nervous system activity was chronically high. An intriguing study, done by the maverick scientists Rein, Poponin, and McCraty at the Institute of HeartMath, demonstrated that a simulated cardiac electromagnetic field increased the growth of fibroblasts activated with growth factors that increase intracellular calcium. What this means is that the *pattern* of the electromagnetic field generated by the heart may influence cell division. Chronic stress, through imbalance of the autonomic nervous system, affects HRV and may induce abnormal cell division that could potentially promote cancer. From a TCM point of view, we note that we are describing a pattern of energy, that could influence every cell in the body. An imbalance in sympathetic and parasympathetic nervous system activity may be a key factor in the regulation of cell division.

The Heart of the Matter: Compassion ☯
and Electromagnetic Field Effects

TCM promotes exercises that balance the HRV, reducing the sympathetic component. According to ancient tradition, anger associated with an obstructed excess of liver yang or Fire can promote cancer. Curiously, Lydia Temoshok, a researcher in mind-body medicine, found that a type C personality that repressed anger, was more likely to develop breast cancer. We now know that repressed anger suppresses our immune response. Could it be that the philosophers of ancient China had a fundamental understanding of the importance of autonomic nervous system balance for health and well-being? Was part of their energy theory an explanation for the influence of the electromagnetic field on cell function? Certainly, many of their healthcare recommendations focused on the maintenance of a compassionate loving heart. Meditation and Qi Gong include the exercises of bringing love into your heart and letting go of anger. This mind-body exercise is called 'metta' or loving kindness, and is well-described in the Tibetan literature. Do we have any evidence from science that we can influence our HRV, and potentially have some mind-body influence over our health outcome? A study by Rollin McCraty and his colleagues at the Institute of HeartMath showed that a technique of compassionate heart-focused meditation (called Freeze-frame™) produced a desired shift in the HRV away from the sympathetic and towards the parasympathetic pattern[13]. The heart rate became more coherent when focusing on the experience of love. TCM theory also predicts that acupuncture should influence HRV through restoring ANS imbalance. Recent scientific evidence has shown that the stimulation of specific acupuncture points influences the pattern of HRV (as measured by a technique called power spectrum analysis)[11]. From what we now know about the influence of the autonomic nervous system and HRV on health outcome (including the development of cancer), techniques to correct the imbalance and restore harmony should be critically acclaimed, and this should be an enthusiastic avenue for research.

☯ *Possibilities, Probabilities and Divination: Genetic Expression and the I Ching*

TCM forms the foundation for a new model of medicine that recognizes a seamless connection between the environment, whole person, molecular components, and a field-effect of energy that communicates between the various levels. Organisms become complex information processing systems. Information is not reducible to single genes. In contrast, genes provide a menu of possibilities, that is various molecular products can be selected according to environmental conditions and the requirement for adaptation. Moreover, as we shall see, the menu of genes itself may be varied when stressful conditions require adaptation. In other words, some genes may produce protein enzymes that encourage mutations to occur in other genes, especially when the organism is subjected to certain environmental stresses. The mutations are caused by enzymes that increase the level of reactive oxygen species (ROS) in the vicinity of the nucleic acids that compose our genes[15]. The ROS require a complex buffering system to keep them in check, but contrary to general opinion, they are not always detrimental to cell function, but play a necessary role in adaptation. A clear example of this is the production of specific immune cells, that are highly selective towards foreign invaders, such as bacteria, viruses and cancer cells. A range of lymphocytes with varying cell surface markers and receptors are produced by 'deliberate' mutation. The appropriate immune cells, that 'match' the foreign invaders, are then selected by a complex process of immune cells presenting the foreign proteins to each other, and then encouraging the proliferation of the selected cells. When the invader has succumbed, the production line of selected cells is normally switched off. If production of a specific cell line continues (which we term a clone of cells), then a cancer of the lymph tissue may develop, that we term a lymphoma. So mutation, which provides new genes that can code for novel proteins, is a normal process of adaptation to the environment. When the system becomes out of balance, then it is the unchecked, continuing proliferation of the cells cloned with the new gene that causes the progression to cancer. A checked system of genetic instability is necessary for adaptation to occur. This mechanism is so flexible and adaptable, that it can be compensated for despite knockouts of single genes.

The coding of protein structures by DNA may be based on a similar system that the ancient Chinese used for prophesy and divination. The system is called the I Ching. It is a dynamical system that initially appears random and chaotic, but underlying its method is a deterministic system of prediction. Its information is contained within an assortment of trigrams, that can combine 'randomly' to form 64 hexagrams. Each component is a digital bit of information, that combines to form patterns that signify different degrees of change and adaptation. The system shares many attributes with the genetic code, as defined by the three bases that form our DNA. What may appear to be a random re-assortment of bases during genetic adaptation may actually be deterministic chaos. A detailed account of the relationship of our genetic code to the I Ching is described in, "The I Ching and the Genetic Code" (see Appendix B).

☯ *Dynamical Systems and Energy-Information Transfer*

The normal function of the body-mind network is a *dynamic* process of communication and adaptation held in check by a field-effect of complex communication between all the hierarchical and heterarchical levels of information processing. Our current methodology for investigating these processes depends on 'snapshots in the dark using a flash', thereby providing a very limited picture and narrow point of view of the communication processes. However, an understanding of this dynamic and holistic system will be necessary if we truly wish to understand the initiation, progression, and control of cancer.

The TCM concept of qi suggests that our molecules do not simply interact in a static 'lock-and-key' manner, but are vibrating with energy that carries information. Transfer of information between transmitters (such as those produced by the endocrine and nervous systems) and cells, as well as between cells, is by vibrating molecules, changes in cell membrane electrical potentials, and electromagnetic waves. The fluctuation in membrane potentials between the outside and inside of cells is associated with the opening of pores that allow the transfer of calcium ions. The pattern of frequency modulation of the electrophysiological potential is like a computerized barcode, specifically signaling to the inside of the cell. In turn, the signal can be transmitted directly to the nucleus, via an intricate structural pipe-work, called microtubules, or indirectly through changes in enzyme activities and intracellular signaling molecules, such as the protein kinases. The information transfer through the microtubules may actually be a quantum event, that is instantaneous, according to some recent theories of cell memory. In addition, part of the holistic information transfer may be through particles of light (photons), suggesting that we may, indeed, be beings of light, as described by ancient Oriental philosophy. The important point is that there is a dynamic communication system between the external environment, via the sensory capabilities of our nervous system, and our genes within the nuclei of the millions of cells that compose our body. In addition, the transfer of this information may be colored by our interpretation of the environment, and by the complexities of cerebral associations and emotional response. Therefore, some information will be tarnished by higher cerebral functions of meaning, a body-mind repository of emotions, and corresponding molecular changes that can influence the behavior of cells.

Disrupted Harmony: ☯ *Chaos and Cancer*

Cancer may be viewed as a multi-factorial complex process, where the harmony of coherence within the field of information processing, has been disrupted, and there is deterioration of its functional integrity. However, a major survival advantage that many cancers develop, is their extremely chaotic growth and function. There is an increase in novel gene expression and mutations, as well as a decreased fidelity in deoxyribonucleic acid (DNA) repair and stability within their genes. This is translated into an extreme variety of cells, in other words a huge menu from which there will likely be some cells that can overcome adverse environmental conditions. That is why cancer can be so resistant to therapy, since no group of cells are the same. If one cell line succumbs to chemotherapy, then there will be another cell line, with different characteristics, that can be selected and will adapt to the new conditions. Therefore, chemotherapeutic war against cancer is usually based on rapid cycling of different chemotherapy drugs, in an attempt to keep up with the cancer cells' adaptation and resistance. Moreover, cancer cells tend to 'want to go and do their own thing'. They have often lost their ability to communicate and cooperate with their previous colleagues in normal tissue. There is a lack of coherence between the renegade cancer cells and the harmonious normal cells. In other words, functional integrity has been lost.

As was previously discussed, the point between order and disorder is the norm. This is the Oriental state of harmony or balance. It is a state of functional homeostasis. The point of balance is not a position of fixed equilibrium, but a dynamic state of readiness for adaptation to change. If the point of equilibrium is entirely appropriate and cohesive with the environmental state, then we call this a system with maximum *fitness*. The system is perfectly balanced between the extremes of rigid order and flexible chaos. We call this point of harmony, the frontier of chaos. This system is poised for adaptation. The process underlying this adaptive system is called a non-linear dynamical system. Environmental change that could signal the need to adapt may include nutritional variation, changes in exercise, environmental chemical exposure, and perceived environmental stress, including psycho-spiritual crises, loss of intimacy and social connection. For bacteria, it is usually environmental nutrition or toxins that require the cells to adapt. However, human beings are much more complex, and many of our stresses requiring adaptation are initially subject to psychological interpretation, emotional response, and behavioral change. This can be communicated to the level of the genes by neuropeptides, hormones, different mixes of immunocytes, and electrophysiological patterns, including HRV. Our environment may be a potent contributor to loss of cell regulation, not only through nutrition and toxins, but also via psycho-physiological modification of oncogene expression.

Is there any evidence that when cancer develops, some normal cells have shifted into a chaotic dynamical system, in an attempt to adapt to environmental adversities? Have they subsequently lost their fitness by discarding their ability to communicate with neighboring cells by contact inhibition? According to Don Coffey, a leading cancer scientist at Johns Hopkins Medical School, some evidence to support this theory of chaos exists[15]. When he measured the cellular motion of cultured prostate cancer cells, he found that they met the criteria of chaotic oscillations.

Psychological Repression ☯ *and Physical Expression*

According to TCM theory, there is no separation between mind and body. If this, indeed, is the case, then we may expect that repression of psychological adaptation and rejection of creative exploration may manifest itself ultimately at the level of cellular adaptation, through the many molecular and electrophysiological processes that I have previously described. This may result in a cell stress or adaptation response, resulting in an increase in genetic plasticity, in an attempt to produce adaptation genes. If the process is frustrated by either physical or psychological paradox, then the system may become over plastic and eventually cell membrane changes occur, resulting in irreversible structural uncoupling from adjacent normal and fit cells. This is clearly not the only reason that cancer develops, but it may contribute to the process. This is not to suggest any blame for developing cancer, any more than we should target fault with our genes, nutrition, or smoking habits. However, it should encourage further research into psychological coping mechanisms and the development of organic disease, plus encourage more counseling resources for supportive care.

God, grant me the serenity
To accept the things I cannot change,
The courage to change the things I can,
And the wisdom to know the difference.
Reinhold Neibuhr

Is there any evidence that psychological profile can influence cancer development? At the current time, this is a very difficult question to answer. The answer often depends on how you measure psychological profiles and what you define as stress. There is evidence both for and against. One study that supports the psycho-physical adaptation theory was published by Lilja and colleagues (*Psycho-oncology 1998; 7: p376*). In this study, the patients' psychological profile was evaluated prior to resection of a breast lump. The patients with the higher grade tumors were found to have extreme emotional reactivity and genuine creativity. According to Temoshok's theory of the Type C personality predisposition to breast cancer, it is the repression of emotional reactivity and creativity that is the critical risk factor[24]. This is further supported by John Astin (*Advances 2001; 17: p142*), who proposes that a positive psychological attitude is when you are assertive and actively pursuing adaptation, *when the possibility for change exists.* However, *when change is clearly no longer possible*, a positive attitude is to let go and accept environmental circumstances. In contrast, a conscious attempt to over-control or, conversely, to be completely helpless, may block adaptation and cause a deterioration in health.

Meaningful expression may catalyze the transformation of a dysfunctional communication network to a non-chaotic and coherent homeostatic state. Beneficial biological changes may be produced by the intimate expression and reception of love.

☯ *Psychological Attitude, Stress, Depression and Clinical Outcome*

There is accumulating evidence that psychological function is linked with outcomes in cancer patients[119-124]. There is evidence to suggest a link between mood disorders and function of the immune system. Indeed, the experience of pain and suffering is intimately connected to immunity.

A mood disorder such as helplessness and hopelessness may lead to a depressed immune system. Treatment of depression and feelings of hopelessness may not only increase quality of life, but may also increase survival[125-127]. In oncological practice, 50% of patients suffer from clinically recognized depression. In 15% of these patients, the degree of depression is severe. Therefore, treatment of depression is an important intervention in the management of the body-mind network of cancer patients.

Treatment of Depression with ☯ Traditional Chinese Medicine

The diagnosis of depression in TCM is complex. Depression may have many different forms with multiple patterns of imbalance, requiring various combinations of herbs and acupuncture points. Studies of the efficacy of TCM versus drugs are therefore mired with methodological challenges. Conventionally, clinical depression is treated with oral medication, such as amitriptyline or the newer serotonin reuptake inhibitor drugs. Studies indicate that acupuncture treatment may be an equally effective alternative treatment modality to drugs in patients suffering from mild depression. In one study, the profile of side-effects associated with acupuncture treatment was shown to be better than amitriptyline[128]. In a single-blind placebo-controlled study of the antidepressant, mianserin, additionally applied acupuncture improved the course of depression more than pharmacological treatment with the drug alone[129]. Since pharmaceutical antidepressants are not usually effective until two weeks after starting therapy, their combination with acupuncture may enable more rapid results with less side-effects.

☯ *Chapter Eight*

Cancer Prevention: Nutrition

- Food for Thought

- The Science of Chinese Nutrition

- Individual Constitution and Nutrition

- Nutritional Correction of Constitutional Imbalance

- Nutritional Re-Balancing of the Organ Systems

- Nutrition, Immunity and Therapeutic Recipes

Food for Thought ☯

Studies of nutrition in the East show that, although total calorie intake of food may be higher than in the West, obesity is relatively uncommon. Why is this so? Genetic factors do not seem to be as important as the type of nutrition. In fact, when Chinese people change their diet to a typical North American diet, the incidence of obesity, diabetes and certain cancers (such as cancer of the colon) increase. Promotion of some cancers can be associated with abnormalities in insulin metabolism, suggesting that diet and exercise may be important factors in the lower incidence of some cancers in the East, such as colorectal cancer.

One important factor is the content of fat in the diet. The Chinese consume an average of 15% of their diet in the form of fat, compared to the American average of 40%. This is still a far cry from the recently recommended reduction of fat intake in North America to 30% of the total number of calories consumed. The Chinese consume about 90% of their protein from vegetable sources, whereas about 70% of the protein consumed by North Americans is of animal origin. Processed carbohydrates, such as sugar, form potent carcinogens when consumed with saturated fats. The fiber contained in the 'undesirable' roughage, which has been stripped from the original food, has major effects on insulin metabolism and prevention of colorectal and breast cancer. The food has also been stripped of essential vitamins and minerals. Unsaturated fats are being replaced in the Western diet by hydrogenated fats, and complex carbohydrates are being replaced by so-called refined sugars.

In combination with a reduction in physical activity, this deplorable diet is contributing to an increased incidence of cancer. Red meat is associated with an increased

To administer medicines to diseases which have already developed and to suppress revolts which have already developed is comparable to the behavior of those persons who begin to dig a well after they have become thirsty, and of those who begin to cast weapons after they have already engaged in battle. Would these actions not be too late?

The superior physician helps before the early budding of the disease.... The inferior physician begins to help when [the disease] has already developed; he helps when destruction has already set in. And since his help comes when the disease has already developed it is said of him that he is ignorant.

Huang Ti Nei Ching Su Wen. The Yellow Emperor's Classic of Internal Medicine

production of cancer-inducing free radicals (molecules that damage the nucleic acids of the genes and can cause cancer), whereas vegetables contain antioxidants (such as vitamin C and E) that can scavenge and neutralize the free radicals, and reduce the risk of cancer. Traditional Chinese cuisine consists mainly of vegetables, with some fish, and only small amounts of red meat. Food is often lightly steamed or stir fried in minimal fat. Partly cooking the food is important since it reduces stress on the digestive enzymes. In Chinese medicine terminology it reduces the stress on the Spleen, which according to Oriental medicine theory, is a major player in digestion, as well as immunity. The increased incidence of pancreatic cancer in the West may be related to dietary stress.

❧ *The Science of Chinese Nutrition*

Green tea (*Camellia sinensis*) and *Panax Ginseng* are two dietary supplements that have been extensively investigated in both the laboratory and in epidemiological studies. Both reduce the risk of cancer induction, and they both may prevent cancer recurrence[90-92]. Green tea contains isoflavones and a powerful antioxidant called epigallocatechin (EGC)[93] (Figure four).

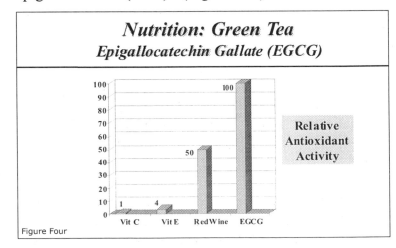

Figure Four

EGC may potentiate the destruction of cancer cells through the process of apoptosis (natural programmed cell death) and by inhibiting angiogenesis (new blood vessel formation that enhances tumor growth and metastasis)[94-95]. *Panax Ginseng* may induce the differentiation of neoplastic cells into normal tissue[96]. Both EGC and *Ginseng* appear to restore normal inter-cellular communication through the gap junctions[41]. Both dietary supplements seem to work through novel mechanisms of signaling and communication through the body-mind network.

The soy bean contains genistein, which is an isoflavone with multiple anti-cancer effects demonstrated in the laboratory[37]. These include the induction of tumor cell death through the process of apoptosis, inhibition of cancer cell proliferation through decreasing the availability of sex hormones, inhibition of angiogenesis, inhibition of tyrosine kinase (involved in intracellular signaling from the membrane to the nucleus), and inhibition of platelet aggregation[97-99]. Some epidemiological studies suggest that populations with a high soy or tofu content in their diet may have a reduced risk of breast cancer[100-102], whereas other studies cannot confirm this link[103]. The phytoestrogens contained within soy may reduce the symptoms of hot flashes associated with chemotherapy-induced menopause[104], although not all studies support this[105]. The isoflavones and phytoestrogens in soy also appear to reduce the incidence of prostate cancer, and may play a role in prevention and as an adjunctive therapy to reduce the risk of recurrence[106-110]. Cell culture and animal xenograft studies show that treatment with soy is associated with inhibition of prostate specific antigen, activation of NF-kappa B (a nuclear transcription factor), induction of apoptosis (programmed cell death), and inhibition of angiogenesis (tumor blood vessel formation)[111-114].

☯ *Individual Constitution and Nutrition*

The best physician looks for the root cause of disease. Then he first attempts to cure it with food. Only if food fails should he use drugs.
Sun Si-miao.
Thousand Ducat
Prescriptions,
Tang Dynasty.

TCM emphasizes appropriate nutrition, according to specific constitutional and disease patterns. In addition, nutrition and herbal therapy is difficult to separate in TCM. Many herbs are used as part of food preparation. Meals are often prepared according to individual constitutions and the seasons, since both can predispose to the invasion of pathogens, and require different interventions. However, in general, anti-cancer therapy tends to produce similar constitutional patterns in various individuals. In particular, there is depletion of Kidney and Spleen qi, and a yin deficiency. Perhaps, not surprisingly, many of the suggested foods are those that we would recommend for a healthy diet today. The only difference is in the fine-tuning of components according to individual personality and symptoms, that may, in fact, reflect our metabolic differences, and should be emphasized more in conventional Western nutritional advice. The 'old wives advice' that beef and barley or chicken soups are good for you if you are feeling sick has stood up to recent scientific evidence. It has been grounded in TCM for thousands of years, since they can tonify qi deficiencies in the Kidney and Spleen. Moreover, TCM has declared since antiquity that, "chicken soup is good for the soul." According to the model of mind-body medicine, this is not a surprise!

☯ *Nutritional Correction of Constitutional Imbalance*

Individual balance is the key philosophy in Chinese nutrition. Your personal constitution defines the appropriate balance of food intake. Our emotions and metabolic function respond to the pattern of food-intake. In turn, our emotional constitution may drive us to eat certain foods that further exacerbate our imbalance. Of course, much of this individuality is derived from our genetic make-up, that defines the pattern of enzyme and molecular receptor levels in our body. However, it may also be culturally determined, and behavior, in turn, can also affect our metabolic function through diet and the mind-body communication network. Thus, what we eat, and our ultimate health outcome is very individualized and dependent on many interacting factors. A TCM history will define the relative excesses and deficiencies in terms of individual constitution. For example, some people are constitutionally dry or yin deficient, complaining of dry feces, dry skin, and a feeling of being too hot. Moistening nutrition, such as honey, millet and milk, may be increased relative to drying foods. In contrast, pathogenic dampness may be indicated by lack of thirst, bloating and indigestion, and a feeling of heaviness. Drying foods, such as adzuki beans and corn, may be of help.

According to TCM theory, food can be classified according to the five flavors: sour, salty, bitter, sweet, and spicy. These correspond to individual constitutions through five-phase theory correspondence that link each flavor to an Organ-meridian system (described in Chapter 10). This is a concept quite foreign to Western Medicine. We can only speculate whether the interaction of food components with our taste receptors corresponds to a more systemic interaction with molecular receptors through-out our body-mind system. One fact, that is pretty well established, is that food does affect our mood states. Hot spicy food may stimulate a cool laid-back personality and aggravate a hot-headed individual. In contrast, the hot-headed person (with an excess of anger or Liver yang) will benefit from cool foods, such as mung bean and cucumber soup. Attraction to specific flavors can indicate the origin of disharmony in the metabolic system. People who crave sweet foods may worsen their Spleen disharmony. The consequence is poor extraction of qi from food leading to fatigue, and a further craving for sweet, 'quick-fix' energy-giving foods. Job's tears, a barley-like grain, can clear dampness, strengthen the Spleen, and help stop diarrhea.

☯ *Nutritional Re-Balancing of Organ Systems*

The Organ systems can become imbalanced. Impatience, anger, and fatigue may be because of Liver energy depletion. A first step is to stop eating food that aggravates the Liver, such as alcohol and sugar. Some practitioners suggest mega-doses of vitamins may be too yang and can aggravate Liver dysfunction. The second step is to eat foods that relax the Liver, such as ginger, small amounts of beef and chicken, congee with mung beans, kelp, turnips and watermelon. Any food which nurtures the Kidney yin (often deficient in patients with cancer) will benefit the Liver, since the Kidney yin is the root of the Liver yin, according to five phase theory. Foods that drain the Kidney energy include alcohol, citrus juices, coffee, milk, raw cold salads, and sugar. Note that large quantities of fruit juice, as prescribed in some anti-cancer diets, may actually be contra-indicated according to TCM theory. Foods that tonify the Kidney energy include adzuki beans, apples, asparagus, bananas, beef and barley soup, brown rice, lotus seeds, small amounts of lamb meat, rosemary, sweet potatoes and tuna fish. In TCM, the body cavities are termed the Triple Burners. This concept is fundamental to the TCM theory of respiration which, not only includes the inspiration of oxygen in the air, but also recognizes the importance of nutrition in the production of energy. When the Middle Burner is impaired, the system cannot extract pure qi from food, and gastrointestinal disorders appear. This is particularly a problem with patients receiving anti-cancer therapy. Symptoms such as indigestion, gastritis, diarrhea, poor appetite, abdominal distension, and fatigue will occur. Patients will have symptoms of Spleen deficiency. The TCM nutritional management includes no ice-cold foods, eating fresh food only, and avoiding dairy products, citrus fruit, millet, raw salad and fruit, salty food, and even tofu. Patients should eat foods that promote the Spleen qi and correct Spleen yang deficiency, and these are often yellow in color. Examples include cooked squash, carrots, pumpkins, rutabagas, and sweet potatoes (yams). Beneficial fruits include *cooked* cherries or peaches, and dried figs. Small amounts of chicken or turkey can be consumed. Spices include ginger, cinnamon, nutmeg, and arrowroot.

Nutrition, Immunity and ☯ *Therapeutic Recipes*

There are some herbs that can be added to food preparations that can increase immunity and help fatigue. Examples would include *Astragalus, Ganoderma,* and *North American Ginseng*. However, the diet should be discussed with an experienced practitioner of TCM, a qualified dietitian, and your cancer specialist, to ensure that there are no deficiencies or excesses, and especially to avoid some rare interactions with anti-cancer drugs. Further details of Chinese nutrition and some delicious recipes can be found in the books, "The Simple Path to Health" and "High Energy Living", both by Kim Le Ph.D. and referenced in Appendix B of this book.

☯ *Chapter Nine*

Symptom Control

- Symptoms of Cancer and Side-Effects of Anti-Cancer Therapies

- The Yellow Emperor's Point of View

- Management of Symptoms and Side-Effects with Herbal Formulae

- Management of Symptoms and Side-Effects with Acupuncture

Symptoms of Cancer and ☯ Side-Effects of Anti-Cancer Therapies

Cancer patients experience multiple symptoms related either to the cancer itself or late treatment side-effects. Even if a patient's cancer were clinically 'cured', the person may still be suffering from late treatment side-effects. For example radiation may cause xerostomia, trismus and skin ulceration. These side-effects have an adverse effect on quality of life, and are often not effectively managed by conventional Western Medicine.

Chinese Medicine plays a useful role in symptom supportive care for cancer patients. Symptoms that can be effectively managed include general constitutional symptoms, such as fatigue and depression, pain, and specific symptoms such as gastrointestinal side-effects and myelosuppression.

The Yellow Emperor's Point of View ☯

Cancer patients receiving chemotherapy usually develop myelosuppression (with risk of infection and bleeding) and gastrointestinal side-effects (nausea, vomiting and diarrhea). They easily become fatigued and develop a reduced appetite. In TCM terms, the chemotherapeutic agents are causing Spleen and Kidney deficiency, leading to a general decrease in qi and blood. Radiotherapy and chemotherapy act as 'heat toxins' that damage the yin and qi. 'Heart fire' is expressed as stomatitis; 'deficient Spleen qi' is manifest as diarrhea. Chemotherapy drugs 'disturb Spleen and Stomach qi', expressed physically as damage to the lining of the stomach and intestines[26]. These

We are healed of a suffering only by experiencing it in full.
Marcel Proust (1871-1922)

69

physical expressions are only part of the disturbance in the body-mind network and will inevitably be accompanied by emotional disorders (such as depression, anxiety and insomnia), and constitutional change (such as fatigue or hyper-excitability and poor concentration). After an evaluation and diagnosis of the disturbance in the body-mind network, appropriate combinations of herbs, acupuncture, nutrition, and Qi Gong may be utilized.

☯ *Management of Symptoms and Side-Effects with Herbal Formulae Systems*

Spleen and Stomach qi are supported by appropriate formulas containing *Rx Ginseng, Poria*, and *Rh atractylodis macrocephala*[26]. Depleted yin leads to dry and sore mouth, thirst, constipation and scanty dark urine. The harmonious relationship between Kidney and Heart is disturbed, leading to insomnia, restlessness, disorientation, palpitations and low back pain. This combination of symptoms is traditionally alleviated with combinations of *Rh Anemarrhenae, Cx Phellodendron,* and *Rx Rehmanniae.* The weakening of qi is associated with depressed immunity and susceptibility to infection and cancer progression. Medicinal mushrooms, such as *Ganoderma, Cordyceps sinensis* and *Shitaki* strengthen the qi, which is associated with an improved immune profile and anti-tumor activity. Another herb with potent immune-stimulating properties is *Rx astragali membranaceus.*

Most patients receiving anti-cancer treatment develop fatigue. This is reflected by inability to concentrate, inertia, and painful exertion. Symptoms of the cancer and its treatment may become indistinguishable. In Chinese medicine terms, both the cancer and its treatment are yang and consume the nourishing yin. Many anti-depressants and some herbal tonics are based on yang, and when

It is highly significant, and indeed almost a rule, that moral courage has its source in identification through one's own sensitivity with the suffering of one's fellow human beings.
**Rollo May
(1909-1994)**

used inappropriately for treating fatigue, can cause major burn-out and sustained fatigue. Many ginsengs are yang herbs and can make some patients' fatigue worse. In contrast, *North American ginseng root (Radix Panax Quinquifolium),* unlike its Asian cousin (*ren shen or Radix Panax Ginseng*) is classified as a yin tonic. It sustains the Lung, Stomach, and Kidney meridians, strengthens the qi, and supplements yin. A major source of *North American ginseng* is from Canada, and it is therefore called *xi yang shen* by the Chinese, which means "root from the Western seas". Patients with fatigue may also be helped by *Cordyceps sinensis, Ganoderma* and *Shitaki,* which are derived from fungi. Interestingly, the same herbs are used for stimulating immunity. This illustrates that abnormalities in immunity and fatigue are related conditions which are represented in Chinese Medicine by yin deficiency, and in Western Medicine by chronic fatigue and burnout. Supplementing the yin may restore the balance in the mind-body system, correcting the fatigue and immune-deficiency.

At least five randomized controlled trials have shown that Chinese herbal treatment can decrease the degree of myelosuppression, reduce gastrointestinal side effects and increase the patient's appetite[59-71]. Importantly, it can also increase the probability of patients completing the scheduled chemotherapy. One randomized trial recruited 669 patients with late-stage gastric cancer[65]. One group of patients was treated with herbs that support the Spleen and Kidney function (*Jian Pi Yi Shen prescription*) twice daily for four to six weeks with concurrent chemotherapy, while another group was treated with the same type of chemotherapy alone. The combined treatment group showed significantly higher immune cell and platelet counts with less general and gastrointestinal side-effects. The percentage of patients completing the scheduled chemotherapy was 95% in the combined treatment group versus 74% in the chemotherapy alone group, a result which was highly significant. Unfortunately, the quality and verification of the data from these studies, which were reported from China, are not at a high enough standard that a definitive meta-analysis can be done at this stage.

In TCM, systemic Chinese herbal treatments and topical herbal applications appear to be effective in treating cancer-related pain. In one study, the effectiveness in pain control was shown to be over 90%[130].

Ginger root has been shown in many clinical studies to have anti-emetic activity[131-135]. It appears to particularly help nausea which may be intransigent to standard anti-emetics. Caution should be used with patients on anticoagulants and those with low platelet levels, since it does have anticoagulant effects at higher doses.

The role of Chinese herbs together with conventional Western pharmaceuticals for symptom control is currently unclear. Laboratory data suggests that they can be effective modifiers of biochemical pathways, immunostimulants, and signal transduction modulators. Potential detrimental interactions and idiosyncratic toxicity are possible. Future studies need to be done using more rigorous methodology and quality assurance. The use of appropriate modeling and suitable evaluative methodologies should enable the integration of Chinese herbology into an emerging model of holistic Western Medicine.

☯ *Management of Symptoms and Side-Effects with Acupuncture*

Acupuncture treatment at acupoint P6 has been shown to increase the anti-emetic effect of drugs for peri-operative and chemotherapy-induced nausea and vomiting[136-137]. Innovative randomized single blind controlled trials have since confirmed these results[138-140] and led to the NIH

(US) consensus statement that, "acupuncture is a proven effective treatment modality for nausea and vomiting"[141]. Stimulation of P6 may be done more conveniently with a small transcutaneous nerve stimulation (TENS) device, such as the Reliefband™, which is worn like a wrist watch (see Appendix A).

Pain is a common symptom of cancer. Causes of pain can be disease- or treatment-related. Acupuncture has been shown to be effective in managing pain and other symptoms in cancer patients[142]. In a retrospective study from the Royal Marsden Hospital (London, UK), 183 cancer patients with malignant pain, iatrogenic pain and radiation-induced chronic ulcers were treated with acupuncture[143-144]. There was an improvement in 82% of the patients, but effectiveness only lasted for more than 3 days in half of the patients. Iatrogenic pain (for example, pain due to radiation fibrosis or skin ulceration) and pain due to secondary muscle spasm responded better than malignant pain. Furthermore, increased blood flow with improved healing of skin ulcers was demonstrated after treatment with acupuncture. I also have similar experience with the high, but short-lasting, effectiveness of acupuncture treatment in malignant pain. I suggest that acupuncture is a useful treatment modality that may best be combined with other treatments to improve pain control, resulting in reduced doses of pharmaceutical analgesics. This has the benefit of reducing the incidence and degree of drug-induced side effects.

Some patients may not be able to access an acupuncturist because of geographic restrictions or poor performance status. A transcutaneous nerve stimulator (TENS) has the advantage of easy self-administration by patients. Recently acupuncture-like TENS (AL-TENS) devices have been developed to mimic the treatment of acupuncture using low-frequency (e.g. 4 Hz), high-intensity stimulation[145].

The goal is to recruit the high threshold type III afferent nerve fibers, that are potent releasers of endorphins. Recent meta-analyses (including a Cochrane Database systematic review) have shown that AL-TENS is more effective than placebo, and improves function more than standard TENS, when treating chronic pain[146-149]. AL-TENS devices are very simple machines that patients can learn to operate in less than an hour's training. An acupoint prescription may then be given to the patient who can administer the appropriate treatments with AL-TENS at home. The Codetron™ is a sophisticated AL-TENS device which has the advantage of reducing tolerance to its analgesic effect, by electronically rotating through a series of random electrical stimulation patterns and acupoint locations.

Recently, at the University of Texas, an electrical acupuncture-like technique called percutaneous electrical nerve stimulation has been proposed to treat pain due to bony metastasis[150]. In this technique, an acupuncture needle is inserted down to the periosteum of the affected bone and another needle is inserted into the nearby soft tissue. These are then electrically stimulated. This has demonstrated promising results for pain relief due to bony metastasis that is not responding to other treatment modalities.

Treatment of Trismus with Acupuncture

LI 4	TW 17
LU 7	SI 19
S 6	GB 2
S 7	

Figure Five

Other symptoms that may be helped by acupuncture include constipation, trismus (post-radiotherapy contracture of the masseter or jaw muscle)[151] (acupuncture points indicated in Figure five), breathlessness[152], radiotherapy-associated proctitis[153], hiccups[154], and dysphagia secondary to an esophageal neoplasm[155].

Suppression of anxiety by acupuncture may be associated with an increase in the pain threshold[156]. Acupuncture may also play a role in the treatment of fatigue and malignant cachexia (body wasting) through the modulation of cytokines and hormones[89,157-159].

Acupuncture Points to Treat Xerostomia

Sp 6	CV 24
St 36	St 5
LI 4	St 6
P 6	

Figure Six

Although the cancer may be in remission after treatment, some patients may still continue to suffer from late treatment side-effects that are associated with a reduced quality of life. Radiation induced xerostomia (dry mouth) is one of the distressing late side-effects seen in patients who received radiation treatment that involved the parotid salivary glands. The presence of this condition renders patients with loss of taste, and difficulty in speaking and swallowing. Recently, acupuncture treatment has been found to increase blood flow to the parotid glands, and may stimulate tissue regeneration in parotid glands damaged by radiotherapy[160-162]. A randomized controlled trial of 38 patients with radiation xerostomia was reported from the Karolinska Institute (Sweden)[163]. Subjects were randomized to either deep acupuncture treatment or superficial acupuncture treatment (using the acupuncture points indicated in Figure six).

The superficial acupuncture group was used as the control, despite previous evidence that superficial acupuncture treatment can have a certain degree of effectiveness and should not be used as a control in acupuncture treatment trials. In this study it was found that in both groups, there was more than a 20% increase in saliva flow rate in more than 50% of patients. In the deep acupuncture group, 68% of patients demonstrated an increase in salivary flow rate. Changes in the control group were smaller and appeared after a longer latency phase. Moreover, patients in the treatment group reported less dryness, less hoarseness, and improved taste. In another study, 70 patients with xerostomia due to either Sjögren's syndrome or irradiation were treated with acupuncture[164]. A statistically significant increase in unstimulated and stimulated salivary flow rate (SFR) was found in all patients immediately after acupuncture treatment, and after six months follow-up. After a review at three years, those patients who chose to be treated with additional acupuncture demonstrated a consistently higher median SFR, compared to those not having additional acupuncture. Despite some limitations in the study design, both studies provide evidence that suggest acupuncture can be effective for the treatment of radiation-induced xerostomia, with minimal side-effects. In a prospective single cohort, visual analogue assessed study of acupuncture in palliative care patients with xerostomia, there was a highly significant alleviation of subjective dry mouth[165].

At the Hamilton Regional Cancer Centre in Canada, we have just completed a phase I and II study of acupuncture-like transcutaneous electrical nerve stimulation (AL-TENS) for the treatment of radiation-induced xerostomia (dry mouth secondary to salivary gland damage). Forty five patients were randomized into three treatment groups receiving AL-TENS stimulation using the Codetron™. The three different sets of acupuncture points were: group A: CV 24, St 36, Sp 6, LI 4; group B: CV 24, St 36, Sp 6, P6; and group C: CV 24, St 5, St 6, Sp 6, P6. The goal of this study was to determine the optimum pattern of stimulation (based on TCM theory) prior to designing a placebo-controlled study. AL-TENS treatment was administered twice a week for a total of 12 weeks. Salivary flow before, during and after treatment was measured, and a survey of the patients' quality of life was assessed. Salivary function was significantly increased and symptoms improved, more so in group A (*Wong R & Sagar SM; 2001; Proceedings of the American Society for Therapeutic Radiology and Oncology*). This study illustrates the importance of selecting the most efficient acupoint combination, prior to doing a single-blind randomized controlled trial.

Acupuncture can reduce the hot flashes associated with anti-cancer hormone therapy. Three prospective uncontrolled cohort studies have been done, one in men castrated for prostate cancer, and two others in women taking tamoxifen for breast cancer. They all demonstrated a reduction in the hot flashes caused by vasomotor instability[166-168]. This effect of acupuncture is through modulation of the autonomic nervous system, and the inhibition of vasoactive hormones, such as follicle stimulating hormone (FSH), vasoactive intestinal polypeptide (VIP) and calcitonin gene-related peptide (CGRP). Therefore, we have both clinical proof and a biological rationale for the effectiveness of acupuncture in the treatment of the hot flashes of menopause caused by anti-cancer therapy.

☯ *Chapter Ten*

Psycho-Spiritual Elements of Traditional Chinese Medicine: Energy Therapies

- Vitalism

- Five-Element Functional Relationships

- Shen

- Spirit and Soul

- Change and Transition

- Chinese Psycho-Physiology

- Coping with Change

- Meditation, Breathing, and Inspiration

- Qi Gong

- Healing and Prayer

- Healing Touch Therapies:
  The Physics of Energy Transfer

Vitalism ☯

Spirituality is the driving force behind the process of life. Meaning and purpose kindle vitality. However the forces that shape vitality are complex and difficult to analyze. This 'life force' is *not* to be found through a reductionist analysis of its components. The answers are *not* to be found through molecular analysis. It is the mysterious complexity of process and function which is the essence of life itself. The concept of energy as an information system, that both drives and directs mental and physiological processes, is suggested by the philosophy of TCM. Restoring spiritual harmony lies at the heart of healing. The restoration of homeostasis of molecular and cell function cannot be differentiated from the harmony of the whole person, including their body, mind, and spirit.

Five-Element Functional Relationships ☯

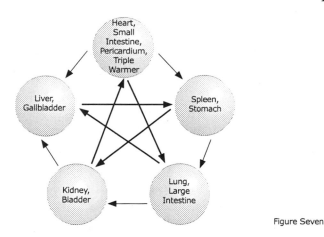

Figure Seven

Psycho-spiritual philosophy plays an important role in Chinese Medicine. It is a complex philosophy based on five-phase (or element) theory (Figure seven). This is a complex system of functional correspondences which integrates body, mind, and spirit. It is an algorithmic representation of communication and relationship processes and should not be confused with physical matter such as organs, tissues and molecules. It represents the transfer of information and, as such, may be analogous to the software of a computer. Fire, Earth, Metal, Water, and Wood are represented in a five-star configuration, with each element corresponding to a yin and yang Organ. For example, the Earth element includes the Spleen (a yin Organ) and the Stomach (a yang Organ). Each Organ is a system which differs greatly from the physiological function assigned to its Western counterpart. Each of the twelve Organs is associated with its own sense, odor, tissue, secretion, season, and emotion. For example, the Wood element is associated with the Liver (yin), the Gallbladder (yang), vision (sense), rancid (odor), ligaments (tissue), tears (secretion), spring (season), and anger (emotion).

Within the five-pointed star, there are two basic types of relationships. These are termed the promotion cycle (*shen* or mother-child cycle) and the control cycle or (*ko* cycle). These are powerful energy relationships, in other words, pathways of information transfer that modulate physiological and psychological function. The *shen* cycle starts as Fire (Heart, Small Intestine, Pericardium, Triple Warmer) and as the mother of Earth (Spleen, Stomach). Metaphorically, fire generates ashes, which produce earth; from earth forms metal, which, in turn, can hold water; water promotes new growth or wood; finally, wood feeds fire, and the cycle is complete. Treatment interventions may be based on an imbalance in this cycle. A deficiency or excess may be in the 'mother' part of the relationship, rather than in the 'child'. For example, an excess in the Wood phase (Liver) will promote an extreme expression of the Fire phase (Heart). Emotionally this may be manifest by anger, tears, sweating, mania, excess arguing, and sleeplessness. Acupuncture to sedate the Wood phase may reduce promotion of the Fire phase and, thereby, rebalance

Ought it to be assumed that in all men the mixture of religion with other elements should be identical? Ought it, indeed, to be assumed that the lives of all men should show identical religious elements? In other words, is the existence of so many religious types and sects and creeds regrettable?

To these questions I answer 'No' emphatically. And my reason is that I do not see how it is possible that creatures in such different positions and with such different powers as human individuals are, should have exactly the same functions nor should we be expected to work out identical solutions. Each, from his peculiar angle of observation, takes in a certain sphere of fact and trouble, which each must deal with in a unique manner.
--William James, The Varieties of Religious Experience, 1902

the emotional excess that would be manifested eventually by physical ill health. The *ko* cycle controls or represses the function of other Organs, as indicated by the arrows that perpendicularly cross the five-element cycle (see Figure seven). Fire (Heart) controls Metal (Lung); Metal governs Wood (Liver); Wood acts on Earth (Spleen); Earth controls Water (Kidneys); and Water controls Fire (Heart). Metaphorically, fire melts metal; a metal axe cuts wood; a wooden tool loosens earth; an earth dam holds back water; and water extinguishes fire. For example, in cancer treatment, hot night sweats and sleeplessness can be a problem. Herbs and acupuncture which supplement Water (Kidney) will extinguish Fire (Heart) and thereby relax and calm the patient.

> The heart has its reasons, which reason knows nothing of.
> **Blaire Pascal (1623-1662) French philosopher and mathematician**

Shen

Shen is the Chinese term for mind. However, it incorporates much more than simply the mind as we know it in the West. It represents spirit, and therefore reflects our vitality and connection to a higher self. *Shen* incorporates consciousness, compassion and intuition. It is based in the Heart, rather than the brain. Bright and shiny eyes indicate strong *shen*. In contrast, loss of spirit and enthusiasm for life (associated with illness) is accompanied by dull eyes. Patients with low *shen* are often emotionally flat and might have a Fire imbalance which can be treated with a combination of Chinese herbs, acupuncture and Qi Gong.

Spirit and Soul

There are also spirits associated with each of the five phases. *Yi* is the spirit associated with the Earth element. *Yi* influences intention, thinking, and empathy. Imbalances can manifest in obsessional thinking and compulsions, and inappropriate emotional connection with others. The

Po, or corporeal soul, corresponds to Metal and deals with vitality, literally the breath and rhythm of life. Past regrets, grief, memories of abuse and trauma and self-worth are all associated with *Po*. *Zhi* is the spirit of Water and encompasses fertility, birth, and maturation. It can exacerbate long-term grudges, jealousy and fear. *Hun* is the ethereal soul which enters the body at conception and leaves at death. During sleep, the *Hun* spirit travels to contact your higher self. *Hun* is fundamental to your life plan and provides introspection and intuition, that are accessed through dreaming and meditation. If *Hun* is not nourished, you may lack direction and cannot make decisions. In making decisions for a program of cancer treatment and care, it is important that your spirits are balanced. Decision-making depends on a balance between intuition and logic. The intuition of mystery and possibility should be balanced with definitive logic and probability. Wisdom is the balance of intuition and intellectual information.

☯ *Change and Transition*

The concept of the five phases is a model of change and transition. Wood and Fire represent the yang phases or yang polarity, whereas Metal and Water are the complementary yin phases or yin polarity. Earth is the neutral balancing point between the extremes. Wood represents incipient growth, a stage of expanding activity, culminating in Fire, that is the symbol of an activity at its peak. Conversely, Metal represents a decline in activity, and Water denotes quiescence. These phases maintain harmony through the described cycles of positive and negative feedback. The five phase system with its engendering and restraining cycles sets out a sophisticated set of systemic relations that

Explore
approaches
which resonate
with your nature,
and seem
intuitively &
intellectually
reasonable to you.
Stephen Sagar MD

describe self-regulation and organization. This concept integrates spirit with the complex inter-relationships at the cellular and molecular level. Indeed, it is a sophisticated model of homeostasis that simultaneously can be used therapeutically at the whole person level, whilst reflecting physiological processes that may be occurring at the molecular level. This idea is both practical and empowering, since it suggests that spiritual attitudes and states of mind may influence molecular processes and health outcome.

Chinese Psycho-Physiology ☯

Corresponding concepts between Eastern and Western philosophies include the mind or *shen* (in the Heart meridian), the intellect or *yi* (in the Spleen meridian), the will power or *zhi* (in the Kidney meridian), the corporeal soul or *po* (in the Lung meridian), and the ethereal soul or *hun* (in the Liver meridian). Balancing of the five elements, associated with these psycho-spiritual concepts, through herbs and acupuncture, may improve psychological and spiritual well-being. Treatments redirect excess energy in one element into another element where there is a deficiency. If there is an excess, it can be sedated. This process of restoring harmony can guide the unbalanced physiology back to balance and restore wholeness or a healthy state. This process starts at the spiritual and emotional level, but may ultimately be expressed at the physical level. The philosophy is well described in the literature[169], but no scientific studies have actually addressed the interaction of herbs and acupuncture with psycho-spiritual adaptation. Some studies of acupuncture demonstrate its efficacy for some patients with depressive-anxiety states, and treatment of these symptoms may have a positive effect on psycho-spiritual transformation and transcendence[128-129]. However, re-harmonizing spirit

Knowledge is the precursor to action, but action is not necessarily the precursor to knowledge. It is a rare case that someone both knows the theory and is able to apply it. If you trust in yourself, then it doesn't matter whether conditions are safe or dangerous. If you are true to yourself, you will not be disturbed by things that happen around you.
Taoist hermit Lieh Tzu, (born 400 BCE)

may correspond to tuning the energetics or informational communication system that connects are psyche (soul) to our physical body. Restoring harmony may contribute to the re-establishment of cell-to-cell communication and may be associated with normalizing cancer growth and contributing to the possibility of cure.

☯ *Coping with Change*

A diagnosis of cancer creates feelings of shock, devastation and awareness of our mortality. It may bring out feelings of regret, guilt, and grief. However, it is also an opportunity for change and transition. It is a challenge that may entail many individual coping skills from 'fighting spirit' to transcendence and graceful acceptance. I believe that there is no single correct approach and that a personal and individual pathway of transition is required. Both individual and group counseling are often beneficial. The Chinese Taoist philosophies of change may be helpful in coping with deep transitions that will occur at the levels of the body, mind, and spirit. Since the Taoist traditions view spirit, mind, and body as a continuum, and not as Cartesian discrete entities, their therapeutic exercises are designed to interact across this continuum. This is in contrast to Western medicine that usually separates the therapy of the spirit (pastoral care) from that of the mind (psychiatry), from that of the body (internal medicine). Even psychiatry has become much more physical in its approach, often utilizing psychomimetic drugs. More enlightened physicians, such as those practicing mind-body medicine, take an alchemical approach, more in line with TCM, where therapy is blended along the mind-body-spirit continuum.

The reasonable man adapts himself to the world: the unreasonable one persists in trying to adapt the world to himself.
George Bernard Shaw (1856-1950)

The Chinese developed a range of techniques involving combinations of breathing, meditation, visualization, self-massage, and gymnastic positions. These were designed to integrate mind, body, and spirit, enable coping with the vicissitudes of life, and to encourage adaptation, both at the whole person and at the physiological level. Breathing was recognized as the fundamental spirit of life. Indeed, the term 'in-spir-ation' reflects the recognition of breathing as a powerful life force. Today, we know that patterns of breathing have a powerful effect on our metabolism and our autonomic nervous system. By changing the way we breathe, we can change our mood, ability to focus, and ultimately our ability to communicate between the mind and the body through our molecules of emotion (such as neuro-peptides) and our immune-response cells. Our state of mind, and our state of body, are both influenced by our pattern of breathing.

Meditation, Breathing, and Inspiration ☯

Fang sung kung is the Taoist term for relaxation breathing and forms the basis of many mind-body exercises. The concept of fetal breathing arose in Taoist tradition. The fetus was seen as 'breathing' through its umbilicus at the energy center of the *tantien*. Therefore, the *tantien* breathing technique mimics this passage of energy flow, intending to restore the health and energy of youth to the body. What we do know, nowadays, is that the digestive tract contains its own sophisticated nervous system, a vast plexus of inter-acting autonomic nervous systems that are communicating with the emotional centers in our brain, as well as our immune-response cells. In other words, deep belly breathing may influence not only our oxygen and carbon dioxide levels, but also affect the way we feel, and improve our immunity. The belly-breathing exercise combines diaphragmatic breathing with a conscious focus and awareness of the breath, recognition and letting go of thoughts, as well as an image of light or energy entering the *tantien* point below the umbilicus. This is a powerful exercise that you can use as a coping technique to enable decision-making through intuition, to reduce side-effects, and possibly to aid in increasing cure through the psycho-immunological connection. A simplified current version is called 'soft belly' breathing.

You can try one form of this exercise, as described in the "Poem of Fang Sung Kung". While lying comfortably and undisturbed on your back, with a pillow supporting your head and legs, focus on your breath. As you relax, imagine the word "soft" while inhaling, and "belly" while exhaling. Gradually scan your whole body, being aware of any tensions, and dissolving them into relaxation, perhaps visualizing a white or golden light entering your *tantien* point on inspiration, and circulating up your spine over the top of your head, through your mouth and down through your heart, into your belly and perineum, spreading out into your arms and legs, and washing away all the tension and replacing it with softness.

The Taoist Poem of Fang Sung Kung

With a high pillow I lie on my bed;
I keep my body comfortable and relaxed.
I breathe in and out naturally.
And say the words quiet and relax silently.
I think of the word quiet as I inhale,
And the word relax as I exhale.
As I silently say the word relax,
I tell my muscles to relax.
First, I tell my legs and feet to become relaxed.
After repeating this three times to get my body at ease,
I tell all my organs and cavities to relax.
I keep my breathing rhythm steady, narrow and even
While focusing my attention on my abdomen.
As my mind enters into a state of mental quietness,
I enjoy this sleep-like but awake state of consciousness.
After I stay in this state for a short period of time,
I rub my face, get up, move around and feel fine.

If you understand what it means to be effortless, then there is nothing you cannot do. You can be yin or yang, hard or soft, short or long, round or square... By knowing and doing nothing, you can know all and do all.

If you do not know how to keep still in this crazy world, you will be drawn into all kinds of unnecessary trouble. You will lose your view of the Way, and, when you realize it, it will be too late, for in losing the Way, you have also lost yourself.
Taoist hermit Lieh Tzu, born 400 BCE

Qi Gong ☯

Kenneth Cohen is a teacher of the Chinese exercise of Qi Gong, which means literally, 'working with energy'. He has developed an exercise called the 'Five Animal Frolics', originally invented by the Han dynasty surgeon, Hua Tuo. This set of exercises mimics animals such as the clawed tiger, monkey and bear. Each represents, alchemically a vital force which strengthens the various Organ systems. The combinations of stretching, gymnastic positions, controlled movement, and breathing, with a concentrative meditation state of mind, can have beneficial effects on the experience of energy levels, emotions, mental agility, and physical strength. In Chinese terms, it circulates qi, prevents stagnation of qi (a cause of illness), improves blood flow, and cnhances the sensation of health.

Healing and Prayer ☯

In both Eastern and Western cultures, different forms of 'hands-on-healing', prayer, and intention to heal through altered states of mind have evolved. The philosophy of Chinese Medicine encourages an appropriate state of mind, such as compassion and healing intent, to accompany a practical procedure such as acupuncture[170]. Meditation is important for both the practitioner and the patient. It induces beneficial physiological adaptations. For example, meditation can restore a balance between the sympathetic and parasympathetic nervous systems[171]. It can also increase melatonin levels that can relieve insomnia, and may have an anti-neoplastic effect[88]. There are currently multiple hypotheses that scientifically support the rationale of healing through influencing the patient's body-mind memory and information system. These include manipulation of the systemic memory system[172], electromagnetic entrainment[16,173-178], interaction with subtle energy[179], and non-local positive intention through compassion and centering[180-181]. Clinical trials of the effect of intent through prayer have shown efficacy in reducing side-effects and complications[182-183], and a recent systematic review and meta-analysis has confirmed the positive effects of 'distant healing'[184].

☯ *Healing Touch Therapies: The Physics of Energy Transfer*

Information can be transferred between the healer and patient. Part of this process may be a non-local quantum event, but recent interest has also turned to the heart and its ability to generate a strong electromagnetic (EM) field, which dwarfs the EM fields generated by other organs, such as the brain. Rollin McCraty of the HeartMath Institute has shown that the cardiac EM field entrains the electrocardiogram (ECG) and electroencephalogram (EEG) of adjacent subjects (*In Pribram, KH. Brain and Values. Erlbaum Assoc. 1998: p359*). The healer must have a focus on love, care, and compassion, a process called centering. The healer's coherent heart EM field entrains the patients's EEG and ECG. This process of entrainment can restore homeostasis or harmony in the patient's unbalanced system through the mechanism of non-linear stochastic resonance. This is a mechanism by which weak, coherent EM fields may be amplified by biological tissue and produce measurable effects in living systems. The effect of the healer on the client is literally a 'tune-up' which rebalances the autonomic nervous system and restores harmony in the pattern of information transfer.

A similar process is seen in the practice of Reiki (from Japan), external Qi Gong (from China), Polarity Therapy

Life is but the coming together of the energies of heaven and earth, and the source of these energies has no beginning and no end. How can one ever possess the way of heaven and earth?
(Taoist hermit Lieh Tzu, born 400 BCE)

and Therapeutic Touch. There is some evidence that they can all reduce the side-effects of cancer and its treatment, and possibly even help to inhibit neoplastic cells[1,185-189]. However, Reiki requires that the practitioner has been 'attuned' by a Grand Master, external Qi Gong usually requires treatment by a Grand Master, and Polarity Therapy requires a long and sophisticated training program. The practice of therapeutic touch requires relatively limited training and may be utilized by the patient's family.

Therapeutic touch was developed within a North American university nursing program by Dolores Krieger in 1972[190]. The practice involves the practitioner laying-on her hands at a short distance from the patient, with a positive and loving intent to heal. The patient's 'energy field' is assessed for the presence of any disturbance, which may be detected over areas of the body involved by disease processes. If an area of disturbance were detected, the practitioner will 'smooth' the disturbance with her hands and channel 'external energy' to heal the patient's disturbed somatic energy field.

Many studies have been done to evaluate the usefulness of this practice. Therapeutic touch can reduce anxiety and pain in dying cancer patients. It can be associated with an objective reduction of biochemical and biophysical indicators[191]. A recent meta-analysis has also suggested that therapeutic touch has a low to moderate positive effect size with an average effect ratio of 0.39[192]. This means that there is good statistical evidence that it can have a significant and important effect on health outcome. Although there are still a lot of controversies regarding the effectiveness of therapeutic touch[193], particularly with respect to technique, end points and controls, the patients' subjective experience should be considered as important since it influences quality of life and immunological status.

Ideally the approach to disease control should be the same in all countries of the world.... Social and economic factors condition not only the incidence and manifestations of the various types of disease but also the extent to which medical knowledge can usefully be applied to their control. Each society must therefore have its own system of medicine and public health suited to its particular needs and to its resources.
René Jules Dubos, 1968

Internal Qi Gong, Tai Chi and awareness meditation are scientifically demonstrated to affect physiological processes, including electromagnetic changes that may represent the flow of qi[185,194]. These techniques encourage a personal sense of control, improve mood, reduce side-effects of treatment, increase immunity, and may be associated with an improved outcome from cancer treatment[195-196].

Further comparative and outcome studies of the various healing touch and somatic meditation techniques are required.

Some exercises to strengthen the meridian Organ systems are well-described in the book, "Chinese Medicine for Beginners", by Achim Eckert M.D., which is referenced in Appendix B of this book.

❧ *Chapter Eleven*

Peter's Story

- An Integrated Care Plan at
  Initial Diagnosis

- An Integrated Care Plan
  at Recurrence

☯ *An Integrated Care Plan at Initial Diagnosis*

Peter had recently retired at the age of 65 years, when he was found to have prostate cancer after his physician discovered a raised prostate specific antigen (PSA) during a routine health examination. He decided to have radiation treatment, knowing the immediate potential side-effects of urgency of passing urine, loose stool, and fatigue. He was also warned that he may develop impotence. His friend suggested that he might wish to visit Dr. Susan Lo for a mind-body approach to coping with cancer treatment. Susan took a detailed constitutional history and examined Peter's pulse and tongue. Peter had been a professor of epidemiology and biostatistics and was an intellectual thinker, often obsessing over detail. He craved candy. His tongue was coated with a thick white layer, and his pulse was deficient in qi, especially over the Spleen location. Susan diagnosed that he had an extremely weak Spleen associated with a history of bloating and intermittent diarrhea. She also discovered that he lacked energy, developed multiple colds, and was intermittently impotent.

Susan suggested a program of nutrition, which included avoiding ice-cold foods, dairy products, citrus fruit, millet, raw salad and fruit, salty food, and tofu. He was advised to eat foods that promote the Spleen qi and correct Spleen yang deficiency. These included cooked squash, carrots, pumpkins, rutabagas, sweet potatoes, cooked cherries and peaches. Small amounts of chicken or turkey were also included, and spices such as ginger, cinnamon, nutmeg, and arrowroot were recommended. Susan also suggested Job's tears, a barley-like grain which can clear dampness, strengthen the Spleen, and help stop diarrhea. She also gave him a recipe for a chicken broth to which he should

Knowing others is intelligence; knowing yourself is true wisdom. Mastering others is strength; mastering yourself is true power.
Tao Te Ching

add prescribed amounts of *Astragalus*, *Ganoderma*, and *North American Ginseng*, to improve his fatigue and immunity. In addition, she prescribed herbs to boost Kidney essence, and implemented acupuncture to tonify his Kidney, Spleen, and Stomach. Peter sailed through his radiotherapy with practically no side-effects.

Following radiotherapy, Susan added selenium, vitamin E and re-introduced some soy products to Peter's diet, following the latest nutritional evidence for prevention. Peter was reluctant to use Viagra™ for managing his impotence because of the inconvenience, and the fact that it caused him to have a headache. Susan treated his impotence with herbs and a course of acupuncture.

An Integrated Care Plan at Recurrence ☯

Several years later, Peter was found to have a rising PSA and recurrence was found in his prostate. His physician suggested an orchiectomy but, although it made sense to Peter, he was uncomfortable with the idea of surgical castration. Susan had recently attended the Comprehensive Cancer Care Conference, organized by the Center for Mind-Body Medicine in Washington DC. She had learned that a herbal combination called PC-SPES was active against prostate cancer and Peter was willing to try this with the cooperation of his physician. Susan Lo discussed the situation with Peter's oncologist and he agreed to monitor the PSA. They both warned Peter about the increased risk of blood clots while taking PC-SPES and his oncologist suggested that he take low dose aspirin each day, and Susan recommended that he should regularly add ginger to his diet, since this also has some anticoagulant effect. Peter's physician suggested regular exercise, and Susan taught Peter some basic Qi Gong exercises to increase his energy levels. He also visits a Polarity Therapist who treats him with bodywork, massage and esoteric energy therapy to restore harmony and maintain psycho-physiological balance.

Peter remains well with a normal PSA and a satisfactory sex life at the age of seventy.

☯ *Chapter Twelve*

Restored Harmony: Life Goes On

- Coping with Follow-Up Visits

- Riding the Dragon

- Traditional Chinese Medicine:
  A Partnership of Alchemy and Science

☯ *Coping with Follow-Up Visits*

After the anti-cancer therapy is completed and you are told that the cancer is in remission, a sense of anxiety and fear sometimes sets in. During the search for more information, the decision-making process, followed by coping with the side-effects, your mind is focused on fighting the cancer and curing it. However, once the therapy is completed, there may be a sense of emptiness. The questions which often arise are: "How do I know whether the cancer has really gone away?" "What tests can be done to detect recurrence?" and "What can I do for myself to enable me to take control and reduce the probability of relapse?"

☯ *Riding the Dragon*

The Tao can't be perceived.
Smaller than an electron, it contains uncountable galaxies.

If powerful men and women could remain centered in the Tao, all things would be in harmony.
The world would become a paradise. All people would be at peace, and the law would be written in their hearts.
Tao Te Ching

Traditional Chinese Medicine focuses on prevention and restoration of the harmony of health. Often, the most important phase of your healing is *after* the aggressive anti-cancer therapy is completed and you are left with that feeling of fragmentation and fatigue. After the diagnosis of cancer, life is never the same again. In a sense, it is a rebirth, perhaps an opportunity to do things differently. The famous psychologist, Lawrence LeShan viewed the diagnosis of cancer as an opportunity for change. Many of the patients who he counseled suggested that they had repressed the callings of their soul. Perhaps for some people, the emergence of cancer was a frustrated attempt at adaptation. What is important is that re-adjustment is required. Some people changed their careers, others took the opportunity to travel and some people changed their relationships. Many people will want to return to their normal routine. That is also just fine, but it is important that you set your boundaries and make it clear to others what your expectations are. Some partners and friends will expect you to be the same as before when you have the passion to change. Others will continue to fuss over you, despite the fact that you may wish to develop your independence. Others may avoid you because of their own fears of cancer. During this phase of further change, it is important to be balanced and to recognize deficiencies in your constitution that may require treatment with combinations of nutrition, herbs, acupuncture, and Qi Gong. The biggest challenge to the practitioner of TCM is to keep people well. Indeed, it is said that in ancient China, the physician was paid to maintain health, and not to treat illness.

The more you know, the less you understand.
Tao Te Ching

Traditional Chinese Medicine: ☯
A Partnership of Alchemy and Science

There is emerging scientific evidence that Chinese Medicine can play an important role in the supportive care of cancer patients. There is enough preliminary evidence to encourage good quality clinical trials to evaluate the efficacy of integrating Chinese Medicine into Western cancer care[197-199]. Currently, the evidence for the utility of TCM in cancer care is promising, but prospective randomized clinical trials for specific clinical scenarios are necessary to obtain reliable and generalizable data. Appropriate stratification and individualization according to TCM diagnostic criteria is possible within the context of a randomized controlled trial[201]. Future integration of different models of health, such as TCM, will lead to further improvement of cancer patients' survival and quality of life. We can embrace an emerging model of holistic medicine grounded with good scientific data. Self-empowerment in healthcare is part of the 'New Medicine'. We are entering a new era of healthcare where the scientist and the alchemist walk side-by-side as equal partners with their patients, integrating the developing technologies with the mysteries of being human.

Give a man a fish and you feed him for a day.
Teach a man to fish and you feed him for a lifetime.
Chinese proverb

Postscript
The Yellow Emperor's Dream

...When he awoke, the Yellow Emperor felt enlightened. He called to his ministers and told them, "I have spent three months in seclusion trying to find out what is the best way to govern the country and cultivate myself. However, I did not become enlightened by trying to think things out consciously. I got enlightened in a dream."

Twenty years later, the Yellow Emperor's kingdom was not much different from the mythical land he had visited in his dream. Not long afterward, the Yellow Emperor left the realm of the living and ascended to heaven, and all the people mourned the passing of a great ruler.

On the islands in the eastern seas are immortal beings who live on dewdrops and pinecones. They do not eat grain, they feed on the wind and vapor, and their minds are as clear and still as the mountain lake. They have ruddy cheeks and they all look like healthy children. They are open, friendly, and have no inhibitions...There is no fear, no anger, no tension, and no dissatisfaction. No one is superior or inferior to anyone else. Everything is bountiful and everyone enjoys the providence of heaven and earth. The sun and moon send a gentle light, the seasons are never harsh, the earth is rich, and the inhabitants are kind. The deities bless the land, and the monsters never go near it. This is the land the Yellow Emperor visited in his dream.

Taoist hermit Lieh Tzu, (born 400 BCE)

Note: Herbs are not FDA approved.

Radio-Support™
Three Treasures Herbs (G. Macciocia)
Contents:
> *Radix Angelicae Sinensis*
> *Radix Polygoni Multiflori*
> *Fructus Lycii*
> *Radix Astragali*
> *Flos Carthami*
> *Radix Salviae Miltorrhizae*
> *Cortex Moutan*
> *Radix Pseudostellariae*
> *Fructus Schisandrae*
> *Fructus Ligustri Lucidi*
> *Rhizoma Anemarrhenae*
> *Radix Paeoniae Albae*
> *Radix Glycyrrhizae*

Chemo-Support™
Three Treasures Herbs (G. Macciocia)
Contents:
> *Radix Astragali*
> *Radix Codonopsis*
> *Radix Oiphiopogonis*
> *Radix Angelicae Sinensis*
> *Rhizoma Pinelliae*
> *Fructus Ligustri Lucidi*
> *Poria Cocos*
> *Radix Pseudostellariae*
> *Fructificatio Ganodermae Lucidi*
> *Rhizoma Dioscoreae*
> *Radix Panacis Quinquifolii*
> *Cortex Moutan*
> *Rhizoma Polygonati*
> *Rhizoma Phragmutis*
> *Pericarpium Citri Reticulatae*
> *Radix Glycyrrhizae*

Suppliers:
www.giovanni-maciocia.com
gmaciocia@aol.com

Distribution (USA):
East West Herbs (USA) Ltd
6400 Hollis Street, Suite 10
Emeryville, CA 94608 USA
Tel.: 1-800 575 8526 (orders)
Fax: 1-510 652 2812

Distribution (Canada):
Eastern Currents (Canada)
#200A-3540 West 41st Avenue
Vancouver BC
 V6N 3E6 Canada
Tel.: 1-604 263 5042
Fax: 1-604 261 8781
E-mail: ec@diablo.intergate.bc.ca
Web site: http://www.acupuncturetcm.com

ReliefBand®
Wrist worn electroacupuncture for nausea and vomiting
Manufacturer: Woodside Biomedical
Tel: (888) 297-9728
www.reliefband.com

Appendix B
Resources

Web sites

- ❂ The HealthWise Connection:
  www.interlynx.net/healthwise

- ❂ Acupuncture Com: www.acupuncture.com

- ❂ Center for Mind-Body Medicine: www.cmbm.org

- ❂ Ralph Moss on Cancer: www.ralphmoss.com

- ❂ Focus on Alternative and Complementary Medicine:
  www.ex.ac.UK/FACT

Books

Comprehensive Cancer Care.
By James Gordon and Sharon Curtin. 2001.
Perseus Books; ISBN: 0738204862

Natural Compounds in Cancer Therapy.
By John Boik. 2001.
Oregon Medical Press; ISBN: 0964828014

The Immune Power Personality :
7 Traits You Can Develop to Stay Healthy.
By Henry Dreher. 1996.
Plume; ISBN: 0452275466

Complementary and Alternative Medicine:
A Desktop Reference.
By Edzard Ernst (editor) et al. 2001.
Mosby Inc; ISBN: 0723432074

The Simple Path to Health: A Guide to Oriental Nutrition and Well-being.
By Kim Le, Ph.D. 1996.
Rudra Press; ISBN:0-915801-62-0

High Energy Living: Oriental Vegetarian Cooking for Health
By Kim Le Ph.D. 1997.
Rudra Press; ISBN: 0-915801-71-X

Stress, Immune Function and Health: The Connection.
Bruce Rabin 1999.
Wiley-Liss; ISBN: 0471241814

The Balance Within:
The Science Connecting Health and Emotions.
Esther M. Sternberg MD. 2001.
W H Freeman & Co; ISBN: 0716744457

Chinese Medicine for Maximum Immunity :
Understanding the Five Elemental Types for Health and Well-Being.
By Jason Elias and Katherine Ketcham.1999.
Three Rivers Press; ISBN: 0609802739

Chinese Medicine for Beginners:
Use the Power of the Five Elements
to Heal Body and Soul.
Achim Eckert M.D.1996.
Prima Publishing; ISBN: 0-7615-0613-6

The I Ching and the Genetic Code.
Martin Schonberger. 1992.
Aurora Press; ISBN: 094335837X

References

1. Macek C. East meets West to balance immunologic yin and yang. *JAMA*.1984;251: 433-441.

2. Schipper H, Goh CR, Wang TL. Shifting the cancer paradigm: Must we kill to cure? *J Clin Oncol.* 1995;13:801-807.

3. Ikemi Y, Ikemi A. An oriental point of view in psychosomatic medicine. *Advances.* 1986;3:150-157.

4. Pert CB, Dreher HE, Ruff MR. The psychosomatic network: foundations of mind-body medicine. *Altern Ther Health Med.*1998;4:30-41.

5.Watkins AD. Perceptions, emotions and immunity: an integrated homoeostatic network. *Q J Med.*1995;88:283-294.

6. Pennisi E. Tracing molecules that make the brain-body connection. *Science.* 1997;275:930-931.

7. Dardik II. The origin of disease and health. Heart waves: the single solution to heart rate variability and ischemic preconditioning. *Cycles.*1996;46:67-77.

8. Song LZYX, Schwartz GER, Russek LGS. Heart-focused attention and heart-brain synchronization: energetic and physiological mechanisms. *Altern Ther Health Med.*1998;4:44-62.

9. Zhang X, Yuan Y, Kuang P et al. Effects of electro-acupuncture on somatostatin and pancreatic polypeptide in ischemic cerebrovascular diseases. *J Tradit Chin Med.*1999;19:54-58.

10. Zhang X, Yuan Y, Kuang P et al. Effect of acupuncture on vasoactive intestinal peptide in ischemic cerebrovascular diseases. *J Tradit Chin Med.* 1997;17:289-293.

11. Haker E, Egekvist H, Bjerring P. Effect of sensory stimulation (acupuncture) on sympathetic and parasympathetic activities in healthy subjects. *J Auton Nerv Syst.*2000; 79:52-59.

12. Rubik B. Energy medicine and the unifying concept of information. *Altern Ther Health Med.*1995;134-139.

13. McCraty R, Atkinson M, Tiller WA, Rein G, Watkins AD. The effects of emotions on short-term power spectrum analysis of heart rate variability. *Am J Cardiol.*1995;76:1089-1092.

14. Lee CT, Wei LY. Spectrum analysis of human pulse. *IEEE Trans.*1983;BME-30:348-352.

15. Coffey DS. Self-organization, complexity and chaos: the new biology for medicine. *Nature Med.* 1998;4:882-885.

16. Cuzick J, Holland R, Barth V et al. Electropotential measurements as a new diagnostic modality for breast cancer. *Lancet.* 1998; 352: 359-363.

17. Thomas D, Collins S, Strauss S. Somatic sympathetic vasomotor changes documented by medical thermographic imaging during acupuncture analgesia. *Clin Rheumatol.* 1992;11:55-59.

18. Chao DM, Shen LL, Tjen-A-Looi S et al. Naloxone reverses inhibitory effect of electroacupuncture on sympathetic cardiovascular reflex responses. *Am J Physiol*. 1999;276:H2127-H2134.

19. Watkins AD. Intention and the electromagnetic activity of the heart. *Advances*. 1996;12:35-36.

20. Jovanovic-Ignjatic Z, Rakovic D. A review of current research in microwave resonance therapy: novel opportunities in medical treatment. *Acupunct Electrother Res* 1999;24:105-125.

21. Riess J, Abbas JJ. Adaptive neural network control of cyclic movements using functional neuromuscular stimulation. *IEEE Trans Rehabil Eng*. 2000;8:42-52.

22. Kosko B, Isaka S. Fuzzy logic. *Scientific American*. 1993;July:76-81.

23. Amkraut A, Solomon GF. Stress and murine sarcoma virus (Moloney)-induced tumors. *Cancer Res*.1972;32:1428-1433.

24. Temoshok L, Dreher H. *The Type C Connection*. New York, NY;Random House:1992.

25. Temoshok L. Biopsychosocial studies on cutaneous malignant melanoma: psychosocial factors associated with prognostic indicators, progression, psychophysiology, and tumor-host response. *Soc Sci Med*.1985;8:833-840.

26. Rosenberg Z. Treating the undesirable effects of radiation and chemotherapy with Chinese medicine. *J Chinese Med*. 1997;55:29-30.

27. Bucinskaite V, Theodorsson E, Crumpton K et al. Effects of repeated sensory stimulation (electro-acupuncture) and physical exercise on open-field behaviour and concentrations of neuropeptides in the hippocampus in WKY and SHR rats. *Eur J Neurosci*. 1996;8:382-387.

28. Dawidson I, Blom M, Lundeberg T, Angmar-Mansson B. The influence of acupuncture on salivary flow rates in healthy subjects. *J Oral Rehab*. 1997;24:204-208.

29. Alavi A, LaRiccia PJ, Sadek AH et al. Neuroimaging of acupuncture in patients with chronic pain. *J Alt Comp Med*. 1997;3 (suppl 1):S47-S53.

30. Cho ZH, Chung SC, Jones JP et al. New findings of the correlation between acupoints and corresponding brain cortices using functional MRI. *Proc Natl Acad Sci USA*. 1998;95:2670-2673.

31. Kerr FWL, Wilson PR, Nijensohn DE. Acupuncture reduces the trigeminal evoked response in decerebrate cats. *Experimental Neurology*. 1978;61:84-95.

32. Kumar A, Tandon OP, Dam S, Bhattacharya A, Tyagi KK. Brainstem auditory evoked response changes following electro-acupuncture therapy in chronic pain patients. *Anaesthesia*. 1994;49:387-390.

33. Zonenshayn M, Mogilner AY, Rezai AR. Neurostimulation and functional brain imaging. *Neurol Res* 2000;22:318-325.

34. Wu MT, Hsieh JC, Xiong J et al. Central nervous pathway for acupuncture stimulation: localization of processing with functional MR imaging of the brain—

preliminary experience. *Radiology* 1999; 212:133-141.

35. Jessel-Kenyon J, Ni C, Blott B, Hopwood V. Studies with acupuncture using a SQUID bio-magnetometer: a preliminary report. *Complementary Medical Research*.1992;6:142-151.

36. Boik J. Emerging trends in cancer research: development of a mechanism-based approach. *Protocol J Botanic Med*.1997;2:5-9.

37. Boik J. *Cancer and natural medicine: a textbook of basic science and clinical research*. Princeton. MN: Oregon Medical Press; 1996.

38. Lao BH, Ruckle HC, Botolazzo T, Lui PD. Chinese medicinal herbs inhibit growth of murine renal cell carcinoma. *Cancer Biother.* 1994;9:153-161.

39. Wang JZ Tsumara H, Shimura K, Ito H. Antitumor activity of polysaccharide from Chinese medicinal herb, Acanthopanax giraldii harms. *Cancer Lett.* 1992;65:79-84.

40. Tode T, Kikuchi Y, Kita T, Hirata J, Imaizumi E, Nagata I. Inhibitory effects by oral administration of ginsenoside Rh2 on the growth of human ovarian cancer cells in nude mice. *J Cancer Res Clin Oncol.* 1993;120:24-26.

41. Kang K, Kang B, Lee B, Che J, Li G, Trosko JE, Lee Y. Preventive effect of epicatechin and ginsenoside Rb(2) on the inhibition of gap junctional intercellular communication by TP and H(2)O(2). *Cancer Lett.* 2000;152:97-106.

42. Baxter LT, Jain RK. Transport of fluid and macromolecules in tumors. 1. Role of interstitial pressure and convection. *Microvasc Res.* 1989;37:77-104.

43. Boucher Y, Jain RK. Microvascular pressure is the principle driving force for interstitial hypertension in solid tumors: implications for vascular collapse. *Cancer Res.* 1992;52:5110-5114.

44. Milosevic MF, Fyles AW, Wong R et al. Interstitial Fluid Pressure in Cervical Carcinoma. Within tumor heterogeneity, and relation to oxygen tension. *Cancer.* 1998;82:2418-2426.

45. Sagar SM, Klassen GA, Barclay KD et al. Tumour blood flow: measurement and manipulation for therapeutic gain. *Cancer Treat Revs.* 1993;19:299-349.

46. Fyles AW, Milosevic M, Wong R et al. Oxygenation predicts radiation response and survival in patients with cervix cancer. *Radiother Oncol.* 1998;48:149-156.

47. Brizel DM, Sibley GS, Prosnitz LR et al. Tumor hypoxia adversely affects the prognosis of carcinoma of the head and neck. *Int J Radiat Oncol Biol Phys.*1997;38:285-289.

48. Lebeau B, Chastang C, Brechot JM et al. Subcutaneous heparin treatment increases survival in small cell lung cancer. *Cancer.*1994;74:38-45.

49. Hejna M, Raderer M, Zielinski, CC. Inhibition of metastases by anticoagulants. *JNCI.* 1999;91: 22-36.

50. Xu GZ, Cai, WM, Qin DX et al. Chinese herb "destagnation" series I: combination of radiation with destagnation in the treatment of nasopharyngeal carcinoma (NPC): A prospective randomized trial on 188 cases. *Int J Radiat Oncol Biol Phys.* 1989.16:297-300.

51. Kleijnen J, Knipschild P. Ginkgo biloba. *Lancet.* 1992;340:1136-1139.

52. Sung WH, Chun JY, Cho CK et al. Enhancement of radiation effect by Ginkgo biloba in C3H mouse fibrosarcoma. *Radiother Oncol.* 1996;41:163-167.

53. Peigen K, Yi T, Yaping T. Radix salviae miltiorrhizae treatment results in decreased lipid peroxidation in reperfusion injury. *J Tradit Chin Med.* 1996:138-142.

54. Sagar SM, Singh G, Hodson DI, Whitton AC. Nitric oxide and anti-cancer therapy. *Cancer Treat Revs.* 1995;21:159-181.

55. Huali S, Shaojin D, Guiqing, Y. Free radical mechanism in enhancement of radiosensitization by SRSBR. *J Trad Chinese Med.* 1994;14:51-55.

56. Zhou Y, Wang Y, Fang Z et al. Influence of acupuncture on blood pressure, contents of NE, DA and 5-HT of spontaneously hypertensive rats and the inter-relation between blood pressure and whole blood viscosity. *Chen Tzu Yen Chiu.* 1995;20:55-61.

57. Stener-Victorin E, Waldenstrom U, Andersson SA, Wikland M. Reduction of blood flow impedance in the uterine arteries of infertile women with electro-acupuncture. *Hum Reprod.* 1996;11:1314-1317.

58. Sersa G, Stabuc B, Cemazar M, Miklavcic D, Rudolf Z. Electrochemotherapy with cisplatin: clinical experience in malignant melanoma patients. *Clin Cancer Res* 2000;6:863-867.

59. Hou J, Liu S, Ma Z, et al. Effects of gynostemma pentaphyllum makino on the immunological function of cancer patients. *J Tradit Chin Med.*1991;11:47-52.

60. Horie Y, Kato K, Kameoka S et al. Bu ji (hozai) for treatment of postoperative gastric cancer patients. *Am J Chin Med*. 1994;22:309-319.

61. Cao GW, Yang WG, Du P. Observation of the effects of LAK/IL-2 therapy combining with Lycium barbarum polysaccharides in the treatment of 75 cancer patients. *Chunghua Chung Liu Tsa Chih.*1994;16:428-431.

62. Ling HY, Wang NZ, Zhu HZ . Preliminary study of traditional Chinese medicine-Western medicine treatment of patients with primary liver carcinoma. *Chung Hsi I Chieh Ho Tsa Chih.* 1989;9:348-349.

63. Rao XQ, Yu RC, Zhang JH. Sheng xue tang on immunological functions of cancer patients with spleen-deficiency syndrome. *Chung Hsi I Chieh Ho Tsa Chih.*1991;1:218-219.

64. Yu RC, Guan CF, Zhang JH. Immune function of cancer patients with spleen-deficiency syndrome. *Chung Hsi I Chieh Ho Tsa Chih.* 1990;10:535-537.

65. Yu G, Ren D, Sun G, Zhang D. Clinical and experimental studies of JPYS in reducing side-effects of chemotherapy in late-stage gastric cancer. *J Tradit Chin Med.* 1993;13:31-37

66. Cheng JH. Clinical study on prevention and treatment of chemotherapy caused nephrotoxicity with jian-pi yi-qi li-shui decoction. *Chung Kuo Chung Hsi I Chieh Ho Tsa Chih.* 1994;14:331-333.

67. Li NQ. Clinical and experimental study on shen-qi injection with chemotherapy in the treatment of malignant tumor of digestive tract . *Chung Kuo Chung Hsi I Chieh Ho Tsa Chih.* 1992;12:588-592.

68. Ning CH, Wang GM, Zhao TY, Yu GQ, Duan FW. Therapeutic effects of jian piyi shen prescription on the toxicity reactions of postoperative chemotherapy in patients with advanced gastric carcinoma. *J Tradit Chin Med*.1988;8:113-116.

69. Chen JZ. Clinical effect of chemotherapy combined with Chinese herbs and Western drugs on leukocytes of gastric cancer patients. *Chung His I Chieh Ho Tsa Chih*. 1990;10:717-719.

70. Lin SY, Liu LM, Wu LC. Effects of Shenmai injection on immune function in stomach cancer patients after chemotherapy.
Chung Kuo Chung His I Chieh Ho Tsa Chih.1995;15:451-453.

71. Wang GT. Treatment of operated late gastric carcinoma with prescription of strengthening the patient's resistance and dispelling the invading evil in combination with chemotherapy: follow-up study of 158 patients and experimental study in animals.
Chung Hsi I Chieh Ho Tsa Chih. 1990;10:712-716.

72. Jin R, Wan LL, Mitsuishi T et al. Effect of shi-ka-ron and Chinese herbs on cytokine production of macrophage in immunocompromised mice. *Am J Chin Med*.1994;22:255-266.

73. Kawakita T, Nakai S, Kumazawa Y, Miura O, Yumioka E, Nomoto K. Induction of interferon after administration of traditional Chinese medicine, xiao-chai-hu-tang (shosaiko-to). *Int J Immunopharmacol*.1990;12:515-521.

74. Feng PF, Liu LM, Shen YY. Effect of Shenmai injection on s-IL-2R, NK and LAK cells in patients with advanced carcinoma.
Chung Kuo Chung His I Chieh Ho Tsa Chih.1995;15:451-453.

75. Zhu H, Zhang J. Treatment of stomatological complications in 31 cases of acute leukemia with Chinese herbal drugs. *J Tradit Chin Med.* 1993;13:253-256.

76. Zhu BF. Observation on 17 patients with radio-ulcer with combined traditional Chinese medicine and Western medicine therapy. *Chung Kuo Chung Hsi Chieh Ho Tsa Chih.*1994;14:89-91.

77. Zhou JQ, Li ZH, Jin PL. A clinical study on Acupuncture for prevention and treatment of toxic side-effects during radiotherapy and chemotherapy. *J Tradit Chin Med.* 1999;19:16-21.

78. Yang J, Zhao R, Yuan J, et al. The experimental study of prevention and treatment of the side-effects of chemotherapy with acupuncture. *Chen Tzu Yen Chiu.* 1994;19:75-78.

79. Yuan J, Zhou R. Effect of acupuncture on T-lymphocyte and its subsets from the peripheral blood of patients with malignant neoplasm. *Chen Tzu Yen Chiui.* 1993;18:174-177.

80. Wu B, Zhou RX, Zhou MS. Effect of acupuncture on immunomodulation in patients with malignant tumors. *Chung Kuo Chung His Chieh Ho Tsa Chih.* 1996;16:139-141.

81. Wu B, Zhou RX, Zhou MS. Effect of acupuncture on interleukin-2 level and NK cell immunoactivity of peripheral blood of malignant tumor patients. *Chung Kuo Chung His Chieh Ho Tsa Chih.* 1994;14:537-539.

82. Liu LJ Guo CJ, Jiao XM. Effect of acupuncture on immunologic function and histopathology of transplanted mammary cancers in mice. *Chung Kuo Chung His Chieh Ho Tsa Chih.* 1995;15:615-617.

83. Wu B. Effect of acupuncture on the regulation of cell-mediated immunity in patients with malignant tumors. *Chen Tzu Yen Chiu.* 1995;20:67-71.

84. Sato T, Yu Y, Guo SY, Kasahara T, Hisamitsu T. Acupuncture stimulation enhances splenic natural killer cell cytotoxicity in rats. *Jpn J Physiol.* 1996;46:131-136.

85. Bianchi M, Jotti E, Sacerdote P, Panerai AE. Traditional acupuncture increases the content of beta-endorphin in immune cells and influences mitogen induced proliferation. *Am J Chin Med.* 1991;19:101-104.

86. Petti F, Bangrazi A, Liguori A, Reale G, Ippoliti F. Effects of acupuncture on immune response related to opioid-like peptides. *J Tradit Chin Med.* 1998;18:55-63.

87. DiPaola RS, Zhang H, Lambert GH et al. Clinical and biologic activity of an estrogenic herbal combination (PC-SPES) in prostate cancer. *NEJM.*1998;339:785-810.

88. Massion AO, Teas J, Hebert JR. Wertheimer MD Kabat-Zinn J. Meditation, melatonin and breast/prostate cancer: hypothesis and preliminary data. *Medical Hypotheses.*1995;44:39-46.

89. Campbell SS, Murphy PJ. Extraocular circadian phototransduction in humans. *Science.*1998;279:396-399.

90. Yang CS, Wang Z-Y. Tea and Cancer. *J Natl Cancer Inst.*1993;85:1038-1049.

91. Kaegi E. Unconventional therapies for cancer: green tea. *CMAJ.*1998;158:1033-1035.

92. Yun TK, Choi SY. Non-organ specific cancer prevention of ginseng: a prospective study in Korea. I*nt J Epidemiol.*1998;27:359-364.

93. McKenna DJ, Hughes K, Jones K. Green tea monograph. *Altern Ther Health Med* 2000;6:61-84.

94. Fujiki H, Suganuma M, Okabe S et al. Mechanistic findings of green tea as cancer preventive for humans. *PSEBM.* 1999;220:225-228.

95. Cao Y, Cao R. Angiogenesis inhibited by tea. *Nature.* 1999;398:381.

96. Lee Y-N, Lee H-Y, Chung H-Y et al. In vitro induction of differentiation by ginsenosides in F9 teratocarcinoma cells. *Eur J Cancer.* 1996;32A: 1420-1428.

97. Li Y, Bhuiyan M, Sarkar FH. Induction of apoptosis and inhibition of c-erbB-2 in MDA-MB-435 cells by genistein. *Int J Oncol.* 1999;15:525-533.

98. Li Y, Upadhyay S, Bhuiyan M, Sarkar FH. Induction of apoptosis in breast cancer cells MDA-MB-231 by genistein. *Oncogene.* 1999;18:3166-3172.

99. Kim H, Peterson TG, Barnes S. Mechanisms of action of the soy isoflavone genistein: emerging role for its effects via transforming growth factor beta signaling pathways. *Am J Clin Nutr.* 1998;68:1418S-1425S.

100. Wu AH, Ziegler RG, Horn-Ross PL et al. Tofu and risk of breast cancer in Asian-Americans. *Cancer Epidemiol Biomarkers Prev*. 1996;5:901-906.

101. Witte JS, Ursin G, Siemiatycki J et al. Diet and premenopausal bilateral breast cancer: a case control study. *Breast Cancer Res Treat*. 1997;42:243-251.

102. Lu LJ, Cree M, Josyula S, Nagamani M, Grady JJ, Anderson KE. Increased urinary excretion of 2-hydroxyestrone but not 16alpha-hydroxyestrone in premenopausal women during a soya diet containing isoflavones. *Cancer Res*. 2000;60:1299-1305.

103. Key TJ, Sharp GB, Appleby PN et al. Soya foods and breast cancer risk: a prospective study in Hiroshima and Nagasaki, Japan. *Br J Cancer.* 1999;81:1248-1256.

104. Scambia G, Mango D, Signorile PG et al. Clinical effects of a standardized soy extract in postmenopausal women: a pilot study. *Menopause*. 2000;7:105-111.

105. Quella SK, Loprinzi CL, Barton DL et al. Evaluation of soy phytoestrogens for the treatment of hot flashes in breast cancer survivors: A North Central Cancer Treatment Group Trial. *J Clin Oncol*.2000;18:1068-1074.

106. Moyad MA. Soy, disease prevention, and prostate cancer. *Semin Urol Oncol*. 1999;17:97-102.

107. Kamat AM; Lamm DL. Chemoprevention of urological cancer. *J Urol*. 1999;161:1748-1760.

108. Adlercreutz H, Mazur W, Bartels P et al. Phytoestrogens and prostate disease. *J Nutr*. 2000;130:658S-659S.

109. Stephens FO. The rising incidence of breast cancer in women and prostate cancer in men. Dietary influences: a possible preventive role for nature's sex hormone modifiers-the phytoestrogens. *Oncol Rep.* 1999;6:865-870.

110. Jacobsen BK, Knutsen SF, Fraser GE. Does high soy milk intake reduce prostate cancer incidence? The Adventist Health Study. *Cancer Causes Control.* 1998;9:553_557.

111. Davis JN, Muqim N, Bhuiyan M et al. Inhibition of prostate specific antigen by genistein in prostate cancer cells. *Int J Oncol.*2000; 16:1091-1097.

112. Davis JN, Kucuk O, Sarkar FH. Genistein inhibits NF-kappa B activation in prostate cancer cells. *Nutr Cancer.* 1999;35:167-174.

113. Aronson WJ, Tymchuk CN, Elashoff RM et al. Decreased growth of human prostate LNCaP tumors in SCID mice fed a low-fat, soy protein diet with isoflavones. *Nutr Cancer.* 1999;35:130-136.

114. Zhou JR, Gugger ET, Tanaka T et al. Soybean phytochemicals inhibit the growth of transplantable human prostate carcinoma and tumor angiogenesis in mice. *J Nutr.* 1999;129:1628-1635.

115. Rabin BS. *Stress, Immune Function, and Health: The Connection.* New York., NY; Wiley-Liss:1999.

116. Jessop DS. Beta-endorphin in the immune system: mediator of pain and stress? *Lancet.*1998;351:1828-1829.

117. Page GG, Ben-Eliyahu S. The immune-suppressive nature of pain. *Seminars Oncol Nursing.*1997;13:10-15.

118. Nutt D. Substance-P antagonists: a new treatment for depression? *Lancet.* 1998;352:1644-1645.

119. Shekelle RB, Raynor, WJ, Ostfeld AM. et al. Psychological depression and 17-year risk of death from cancer. *Psychosomatic medicine.*1981;43:117-125.

120. Levy SM, Wise BD. Psychosocial risk factors, natural immunity, and cancer progression: implications for intervention. *Current Psychological Research and Reviews.*1987;6:229-243.

121. Ramirez AJ, Craig TKJ, Watson JP, et al. Stress and relapse of breast cancer. *Br Med J.* 1989;298:291-293.

122. Andersen BL, Farrar WB, Golden-Kreutz D, et al. Stress and immune responses after surgical treatment of regional breast cancer. *J Natl Cancer Inst.*1998.90:30-36.

123. Orsi AJ, McCorkle R, Tax AW et al. The relationship between depressive symptoms and immune status phenotypes in patients undergoing surgery for colorectal cancer. *Psycho-Oncology.*1996;5:311-319.

124. Watson M, Haviland JS, Greer S, Davidson J, Bliss JM. Influence of psychological response on survival in breast cancer: a population-based cohort study. *Lancet.*1999;354:1331-1336.

125. Fawzy FI. Psychosocial interventions for patients with cancer: what works and what doesn't. *Eur J Cancer.*1999;35:1559-1564.

126. Fawzy FI, Fawzy NW, Arndt LA, Pasnau R. Critical review of psychosocial interventions in cancer care. *Arch Gen Psychiatry.*1995;52:100-113.

127. Spiegel D, Bloom JR, Kraemer HC, Gottheil E. Effect of psychosocial treatment on survival of patients with metastatic breast cancer. *Lancet*. 1989;ii:888-891.

128. Han JS. Electroacupuncture: an alternative to antidepressants for treating affective diseases. *Intern J Neuroscience*. 1986;29: 79-92.

129. Roschke J, Wolf C, Muller MJ et al. The benefit from whole body acupuncture in major depression. *J Affect Disord* 2000;57:73-81.

130. Yang G, Liu J, Xie J, et al. Controlling cancerous pain with analgesic powders for cancers. *J Tradit Chin Med*. 1995;15:174-177.

131. Fischer-Rasmussen W, Kjaer SK, Dahl C, Asping U. Ginger treatment of hyperemesis gravidarum. *Eur J Obstet Gynecol Reprod Biol*. 1991;38:19-24.

132. Bone ME, Wilkinson DJ, Young JR, McNeil J, Charlton S. Ginger root-a new antiemetic: The effect of ginger root on postoperative nausea and vomiting after major gynaecological surgery. *Anaesthesia*. 1990;45:669-671.

133. Mowrey DB, Clayson DE. Motion sickness, ginger, and psychophysics. *Lancet*. 1982;i:655-657.

134. Grontved A, Hentzer E. Vertigo-reducing effects of ginger root. A controlled clinical study. *J Otorhinolaryngol Relat Spec*. 1986;48:282-286.

135. Grontved A, Brask T, Kambskard J, Hentzer E. Ginger root against seasickness.: A controlled trial on the open sea. *Acta Otolaryngol*. 1988;195:45-49.

136. Dundee JW, Chestnutt WN, Ghaly RG, Lynas AGA. Traditional Chinese acupuncture: a potentially useful antiemetic? *BMJ*.1986;293:583-584.

137. Dundee JW, Ghaly RG, Fitzpatrick KTJ Abram WP, Lynch GA. Acupuncture prophylaxis of cancer chemotherapy-induced sickness. *J Royal Soc Med.* 1989;82:268-271.

138. Al-Sadi M, Newman B, Julious SA. Acupuncture in the prevention of postoperative nausea and vomiting. *Anaesthesia.* 1997;52:658-661.

139. Schlager A, Offer, T, Baldissera I. Laser stimulation of acupuncture point P6 reduces postoperative vomiting in children undergoing strabismus surgery. *Brit J Anaesthesia.* 1998;81:529-532.

140. Lee A. Done ML. The use of nonpharmacologic techniques to prevent postoperative nausea and vomiting: a meta-analysis. *Anesth Analg.* 1999;88:1362-1369.

141. NIH Consensus Development Panel on Acupuncture. Acupuncture. *JAMA.* 1998;280:1518-1524.

142. Thompson JW, Filshie J. Transcutaneous electrical nerve stimulation (TENS) and acupuncture. In Doyle D, Hanks GWC, MacDonald (eds). *Oxford Textbook of Palliative Medicine (second edition).* Oxford, UK; Oxford University Press: 1998.

143. Filshie J, Redman D. Acupuncture and malignant pain problems. *Eur J Surg Oncol.* 1985;11:389-394.

144. Filshie J. Acupuncture for malignant pain. *Acupuncture in Medicine.*1984;May:12-14.

145. Pomeranz B, Niznik G. Codetron: a new electrotherapy device overcomes the habituation problems of conventional TENS devices. *Am J Electromed* 1987;2:22-26.

146. Patel M, Gutzwiller F, Paccaud F, Marazzi A. A meta-analysis of acupuncture for chronic pain. *Int J Epidemiol.* 1989;18:900-906.

147. Ernst E, White AR. Acupuncture for back pain: a meta-analysis of randomized controlled trials. *Arch Intern Med.* 1998;158:2235-2241.

148. Ghoname E-S, Craig WF, White PF, et al. Percutaneous electrical nerve stimulation for low back pain: A randomized crossover study. *JAMA.* 1999;281:818-823.

149. Gadsby JG, Flowerdew MW. Review: transcutaneous electrical nerve stimulation reduces pain and improves range of movement in chronic low-back pain. *Evidence-Based Medicine.* 1997;July/Aug:107.

150. Ahmed HE, Craig WF, White PF et al. Percutaneous electrical nerve stimulation (PENS): a complementary therapy for the management of pain secondary to bony metastasis. *Clin J Pain* 1998;14:320-323.

151. Ernst E, White AR. Acupuncture as a treatment for temporomandibular joint dysfunction: A systematic review of randomized trials. *Arch Otolaryngol Head Neck Surg.* 1999;125:269-272.

152. Filshie J, Penn K, Ashley S et al. Acupuncture for the relief of cancer-related breathlessness. *Palliative Medicine.* 1996;10:145-150.

153. Zhang, Z. Effect of acupuncture on 44 cases of radiation rectitis following radiation therapy for carcinoma of the cervix uteri. *J Tradit Chinese Med.* 1987;7:139-140.

154. Yan L. Treatment of persistent hiccupping with electro-acupuncture at "hiccup-relieving" point. *J Traditl Chinese Med.* 1988;8:29-30.

155. Feng R. Relief of oesophageal carcinomatous obstruction by acupuncture. *J Tradit Chinese Med.* 1984;4:3-4.

156. Widerstrom-Noga E, Dyrehag LE, Borglum-Jensen L, et al. Pain threshold responses to two different modes of sensory stimulation in patients with orofacial muscular pain: Psychological considerations. *J Orofac Pain.* 1998;12:27-34

157. Glaus A. Fatigue and cachexia in cancer patients. *Support Care Cancer.*1998; 6:77-78.

158. Stone P, Richards M, Hardy J. Fatigue in patients with cancer. *Eur J Cancer.*1998;34:1670-1676.

159. Lissoni P, Paulorossi F, Tancini G et al. Is there a role for melatonin in the treatment of neoplastic cachexia? *Eur J Cancer.*1996;32A:1340-1343.

160. Blom M, Dawidson I, Angmar-Mansson B. The effect of acupuncture on salivary flow rates in patients with xerostomia. *Oral Surg Oral Med Oral Pathol.* 1992;73:293-298.

161. Talal N, Quinn JH, Daniels TE. The clinical effects of electrostimulation on salivary function of Sjögrens syndrome patients: A placebo controlled study. *Rheumatol Int.* (1992);12:43-45.

162. Blom M, Lundeberg T, Dawidson I, Angmar-Mansson B. Effects on local blood flux of acupuncture stimulation used to treat xerostomia in patients suffering from Sjögren's syndrome. *J Oral Rehab.* 1993;20:541-548.

163. Blom M, Dawidson I, Fernberg J-O, Johnson G, Angmar-Mansson B. Acupuncture treatment of patients with radiation-induced xerostomia. *Oral Oncol, Eur J Cancer.* 1996; 32B:182-190.

164. Blom M, Lundeberg T. Long-term follow-up of patients treated with acupuncture for xerostomia and the influence of additional treatment. *Oral Dis.* 2000;6:15-24.

165. Rydholm M, Strang, P. Acupuncture for patients in hospital-based home care suffering from xerostomia. *J Pall Care.* 1999:15:20-23.

166. Hammar M, Frisk J, Grimas, O. Acupuncture treatment of vasomotor symptoms in men with prostatic carcinoma: A pilot study. *J Urol.* 1999;161:853-856.

167. Cumins SM, Brunt AM. Does acupuncture influence the vasomotor symptoms experienced by breast cancer patients taking tamoxifen? *Acupunct in Med.* 2001;18:28-29.

168. Tukmachi E. Treatment of hot flushes in breast cancer patients with acupuncture. *Acupunct in Med.* 2000;18:22-27.

169. Hammer L. *Dragon Rises; Red Bird Flies: Psychology, Energy and Chinese Medicine.* 1990. Station Hill Press; Barrytown NY.

170. Rapgay L, Rinpoche VL, Jessum R. Exploring the nature and functions of the mind: a Tibetan Buddhist meditative perspective. *Prog Brain Res*. 2000;122:507-515.

171. Benson H. *The Relaxation Response*. New York, NY: 1975.

172. Schwartz GER, Russek, LGS. *The Living Energy Universe*. Charlottesville, VA; Hampton Roads:1999.

173. Childre D, Cryer B. *From Chaos to Coherence*. Boston, MA; Butterworth-Heinemann:1999.

174. Benford MS, Talnagi J, Doss DB, Boosey, S, Arnold LE. Gamma radiation fluctuations during alternative healing therapy. *Altern Ther Health Med*. 1999;5:51-56.

175. Seto A, Kusaka C, Nakazato S, et al. Detection of extraordinary large bio-magnetic field strength from human hand. *Acupunct Electro Ther Res Inst J*. 1992;17:75-94.

176. Zimmerman J. Laying-on-of-hands healing and therapeutic touch: a testable theory. *BEMI Currents J Bioelectromagnetics Inst*.1990;2:8-17.

177. Sisken BF, Walder J. Therapeutic aspects of electromagnetic fields for soft tissue healing. In: Blank M, ed. *Electromagnetic fields: Biological interactions and mechanisms. Advances in Chemistry Series*. 1995:277-285.

178. Walleczek J. Electromagnetic field effects on cells of the immune system: the role of calcium signalling. *FASEB J*. 1992;6:3177-3185.

179. Tiller WA, Pecci EF. *Science and Human Transformations: Subtle Energies, Intentionality and Consciousness.* Walnut Creek, CA; Pavior: 1997.

180. Nadeau R, Kafatos M. *The Non-Local Universe: The New Physics and Matters of the Mind.* Oxford, UK: Oxford University Press: 2000.

181. Grinberg-Zylberbaum J, Delaflor M, Attie L, Goswami A. The Einstein-Podolsky-Rosen paradox in the brain: the transferred potential. *Physics Essays.*1994;4:422-428.

182. Dossey L. Healing Words: *The Power of Prayer and the Practice of Medicine.* San Francisco; HarperSanFrancisco:1995.

183. Harris WS, Gowda M, Kolb JW et al. A randomized, controlled trial of the effects of remote, intercessory prayer on outcomes in patients admitted to the coronary care unit. *Arch Intern Med.* 1999;159:2273-2278.

184. Astin JA, Harkness E, Ernst E. The efficacy of "distant healing": a systematic review of randomized trials. *Ann Intern Med* 2000;132:903-910.

185. Cohen KS. *The way of Qigong: The art and science of Chinese energy healing.* New York, NY; Ballantine: 1997.

186. Quizi S, Li Z. A clinical observation of Qigong as a therapeutic aid for advanced cancer patients (abstract). *First World Conference for Academic Exchange of Medical Qigong;* Beijing;1988.

187. Feng L, Juqing Q, Shugine C. A study of the effect of the emitted qi of Qigong on human carcinoma cells (abstract). *First World Conference for Academic Exchange of Medical Qigong;* Beijing;1988.

188. Olson K, Hanson J. Using Reiki to manage pain: a preliminary report. *Cancer Prevention & Control.* 1997;1:108-113.

189. Shah S, Ogden AT, Pettker CM et al. A study of energy healing on in vitro tumor cell proliferation. *J Alt Comp Med.* 1999;5:359-365.

190. Horrigan B. Dolores Krieger RN, PhD: Healing with therapeutic touch. *Altern Ther Health Med.*1998;4:87-92.

191. Cox C, Hayes J. Physiologic and psychodynamic responses to the administration of therapeutic touch in critical care. *Complement Ther Nurs Midwifery.* 1999;5:87-92.

192. Winstead-Fry P, Kijek J. An integrative review and meta-analysis of therapeutic touch research. *Altern Ther Health Med.*1999;5:58-62.

193. Rosa l, Rosa E, Sarner L, Barrett S. A close look at therapeutic touch. *JAMA.*1998;279:1005-1008.

194. Syldona M, Rein G. The use of DC electrodermal potential measurements and healer's felt sense to assess the energetic nature of qi. *J Alt Comp Med.* 1999;5:329-347.

195. Young DR, Appel LJ, Jee SH, Miller ER. The effects of aerobic exercise and T'ai Chi on blood pressure in older people: results of a randomized trial. *J Am Geriatr Soc.* 1999; 47:277-284.

196. Meares A. Regression of osteogenic sarcoma metastases associated with intensive meditation. *Med J Aust.*1978;2:433.

197. Sagar SM. Unproven Cancer Therapies. *Annals of the Royal College of Physicians and Surgeons of Canada.* 1998; 31:160.

198. Sagar SM. *Alternative views on alternative therapies. CMAJ.*1999;160:1697-1698.

199. Tagliaferri M, Cohen I, Tripathy D. Complementary and alternative medicine in early-stage breast cancer. *Semin Oncol.* 2001;28:121-134.

200. Fontanarosa PB, Lundberg GD. Alternative medicine meets science. *JAMA.* 1998. 280:1618-1619.

201. Bensoussan A, Talley NJ, Hing M, et al. Treatment of irritable bowel syndrome with chinese herbal medicine: A randomized controlled trial. *JAMA.* 1998.280:1585-1589.

Index

A

abdominal distension, 67
abuse and trauma, 82
acid-base balance, 9
Acquired Immunodeficiency Disease Syndrome (AIDS), 37
acupuncture and acupressure points, 7-8, 10, 12-15, 19-20, 22-23, 29, 31, 35, 39-41, 46, 48, 51, 59, 70, 72-77, 80-81, 83, 87, 93, 97

  CV24, 77
  GB39, 41
  GV14, 41
  LI4, 40, 77
  LI 11, 40
  P6, 7, 12, 41, 72-73, 77
  Sp6, 41
  Sp10, 41
  St5, 77
  St6, 77
  St36, 41, 77
  UB20, 41

acupuncture-like transcutaneous nerve stimulation (AL-TENS), 73-74, 76-77
adaptation, 52-54, 56-58, 83, 85, 87, 96
addiction, 21
adrenal gland, 45
adrenocortical trophic hormone (ACTH), 45
afferent peripheral nerves, 23, 49, 74
alchemy, 27
alcohol, 66
alternative healthcare system, 26
amitriptyline, 59
anti-thrombotic, 33
ancient wisdom, 27
anesthesia, 13
anger, 3, 14, 21, 51, 65-66, 80, 98

angiogenesis, 63
anti-androgen, 42
anticoagulants, 34, 72
antidepressants, 59
anti-emetic, 72
anti-inflammatory, 32, 40
antioxidant, 32, 62
anti-tumor activity, 32, 70
anxiety, 3, 12-13, 47, 70, 75, 83, 89, 96
apoptosis, 33, 63
appetite, 10, 14-15, 67, 69, 71
art (of healing), 27
aspirin, 93
assertive, 58
Astin, John, 58
astral energy, 27
autonomic nervous system, 5, 9-10, 19-20, 23, 49-52, 77, 85, 88
autopoietic, 19
awareness, 4, 48, 84
  meditation, 90
  of the breath, 85

B

back pain, 70
Bacon, Francis, 4
balance, 8-10, 19-22, 26, 31-33, 35, 39, 41, 46-51, 53, 56, 64, 71, 82-83, 87, 94
barcode, 54
bark, 32
basal ganglia, 48
BCG, 39
beat-to-beat variation of the heart, 6, 10, 49
beliefs, 27
Bienenstock, John, 45
biological response, 25
bladder cancer, 39
bleeding, 69
blood, 10, 20, 33-34, 40-41, 46, 63, 69
blood clots, 93

blood flow, 5, 9-10, 31, 33-35, 48, 73, 75-76
body-mind communication network, 18-19, 39
bone metastasis, 74
brain stem, 5, 22, 44, 48
breast cancer, 21, 51, 58, 61, 63, 77
breathing, 9, 85-87
  breathing exercises, 14
  breathing, meditation, 84
  breathlessness, 75
Buddhists, 6
buffering system, 52
burn-out, 26, 46, 71

C

cachexia, 75
Calcitonin Gene Related Peptide (CGRP), 77
calcium ions, 54
cancer cells, 18, 31-33, 37-40, 47, 52, 56-57, 63
cancer-killing, 31, 39
cancer of the colon, 61
carcinogens, 61
cardiovascular disease, 3
cell,
  behavior, 6
  contact, 33
  division, 33, 49-50
  membranes, 4, 31
  proliferation, 5, 9, 63
  communication, 38, 47, 84
centering, 6, 88
cervix cancer, 38
c-fes (oncogene), 46
chakras, 27
change and transition, 82, 84
chaos, 53, 56-57
chemical exposure, 56
chemical reactions, 27, 37
Chemo-Support™, 15, 22

About the Author

Stephen M. Sagar
BSc(hons), MB BS, MRCP, FRCR, FRCPC

Dr Sagar trained as a physician in London, England and now lives in Canada. He is a cancer specialist in clinical practice at the Hamilton Regional Cancer Centre and at the Canadian Radiation Oncology Services in Toronto.

Dr Sagar trained in acupuncture with the Acupuncture Foundation of Canada and was a founding director of the Complementary Medicine section of the Ontario Medical Association.

He has a university appointment as Associate Professor in the Department of Medicine at McMaster University, where he teaches complementary medicine, spirituality, and supportive care for many courses. He has been an examiner for the Royal College of Physicians and Surgeons of Canada, and is currently a member of the teaching faculty at the Center for Mind-Body Medicine, and a member of the planning committee for the annual Comprehensive Cancer Care conference in Washington DC.

He is an educator for many international courses on complementary medicine and spirituality, including teaching the role of complementary medicine in clinical practice for oncologists at the annual ASTRO meeting.

His research interests include new models of healthcare, mind-body medicine, complementary medicine, and spirituality.

He is on the international editorial board of the evidence-based journal, Focus on Alternative and Complementary Therapies (FACT).

Dr Sagar may be contacted to arrange speaking engagements through DreamingDragonFly Communications™
Email address: dragonflycom@home.com.